the 5:2 diet
recipe book

This book was created by Bounty Books based on
materials licensed to it by Bauer Media Books, Sydney

Bauer Media Limited
54 Park Street, Sydney
GPO Box 4088, Sydney, NSW 2001
www.awwcookbooks.com.au

Published in 2013 by Bounty Books,
a division of Octopus Publishing Group Ltd
Endeavour House, 189 Shaftesbury Avenue
London WC2H 8JY
www.octopusbooks.co.uk
Reprinted 2014 (twice)

An Hachette UK Company
www.hachette.co.uk

ISBN 978-0-753726-06-8

Printed and bound in China

Publisher: Samantha Warrington
Editorial and Design Manager: Gary Almond
Food Director: Pamela Clark
Editor: Jane Birch
Designer: Chris Bell/cbdesign

the 5:2 diet recipe book

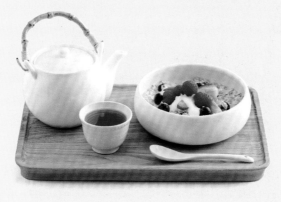

Bounty
BOOKS

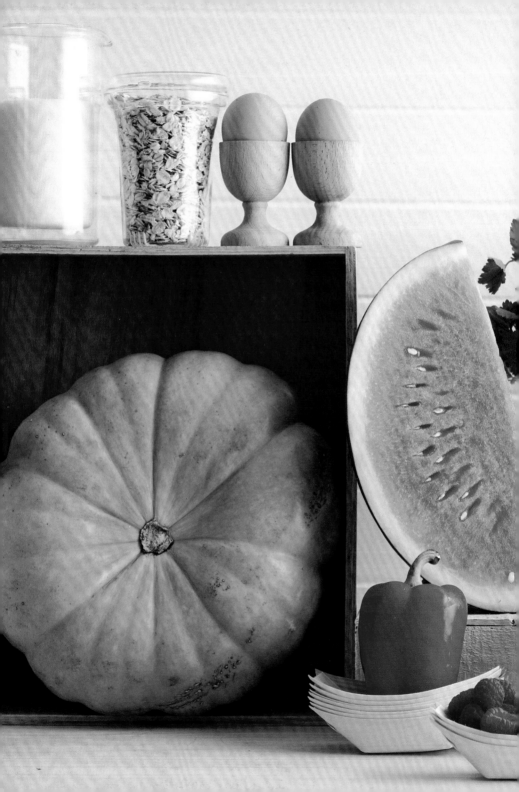

contents

The 5:2 diet explained   6

Breakfasts   14

Snacks   34

Lunches & light meals   40

Mains   76

Desserts   116

Index   140

Conversion charts   143

The 5:2 diet explained

The weight-loss plan that everyone's talking about, the 5:2 diet is a safe, effective and amazingly simple way to lose weight and benefit your health at the same time. And it's the only diet that allows you to enjoy traditionally banned treats such as pizza and chocolate!

How it works

The 5:2 diet is based on the concept of intermittent fasting; it allows normal eating, including treats and meals out, for five days a week and then restricts calories for the other two days. Women are allowed 500 calories per day on fasting days and men 600 calories a day.

Feast and famine

There's nothing new about fasting; all the major religions, including Judaism, Christianity, Buddhism and Islam, embrace it for spiritual wellbeing. And our ancestors – cavemen and hunter-gatherers – would have had periods of famine, when they subsisted on berries, roots and leaves, followed by feasting when an animal was killed.

Our bodies, despite the never-ending opportunities to eat (and to over-eat) that modern Western life offers, are still designed to expect food to be scarce sometimes and more plentiful at others, which is why many scientists believe that intermittent fasting could be a particularly good way to keep slim and fight ageing.

Particular research interest is currently focused on a hormone called IGF-1, or insulin-like growth factor. IGF-1 is important for growth when we are young but, for adults, lower levels of IGF-1 are linked to a decreased cancer risk. Researchers think that the repeated pattern of on/off fasting that is the key to the 5:2 diet might help to keep IGF-1 at persistently low and healthy levels.

The health benefits

When you eat only 500 or 600 calories for two days a week and don't significantly overcompensate on the remaining five days (as evidence shows most people don't), it stands to reason that you will lose weight. Research is still ongoing into the subject of intermittent fasting but there is evidence of other health benefits in addition to weight loss and the improved health that comes with that.

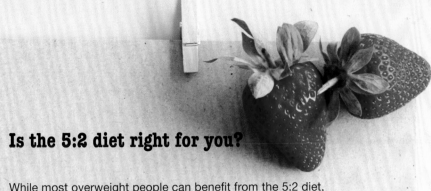

Is the 5:2 diet right for you?

While most overweight people can benefit from the 5:2 diet, some should avoid it:

- children and adolescents
- pregnant and breastfeeding women and women trying to get pregnant
- people with a body mass index (BMI) of 20 or less
- athletes or those in training for a big marathon or other stamina event
- people who have diabetes
- those with irritable bowel syndrome
- anyone who has been diagnosed with an eating disorder, either recently or in the past

Check with your doctor if you are at all uncertain about whether this diet is right for you.

Fasting day calories

- women should have no more than 500 calories
- men should have no more than 600 calories

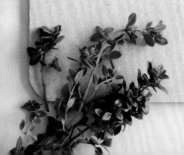
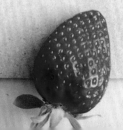

Research published in the *Journal of Nutritional Biochemistry* showed that feeding rats and mice only every other day improved the health and function of their brains, hearts and other organs while other studies have shown that mice and rats on intermittent fasts develop fewer cancers, are less prone to neurological disorders and live 30 per cent longer than rodents that are fed every day.

Brain function

Much of the research into intermittent fasting began with, and continues to focus on, healthy ageing and brain ageing specifically. Findings from the National Institute on Aging in the United States revealed that rats and mice that have been genetically engineered to develop Alzheimer's disease were much slower to do so if put on an intermittent fasting regime than those rodents on a normal diet.

Diabetes and blood sugar control

Any weight loss in obese people, no matter how they go about doing it, will usually result in the body becoming more sensitive to insulin which is an important step in reducing the risk of developing diabetes. In study at Manchester's Wynthenshawe Hospital, women on a 5:2-style diet were compared with women restricted to a daily intake of 1,500 calories. Both groups lost weight and reduced their cholesterol levels and blood pressure but those in the 5:2 diet group also showed signs of decreased diabetes risk.

Heart disease

A reduction in cardiovascular risk factors – for example 'bad' (LDL) cholesterol and high blood pressure – can be expected if you follow the 5:2 diet. Much of the research in this area, done at the University of Illinois at Chicago, confirms the benefit that intermittent fasting has for a healthy heart.

Fasting days

The beauty of the 5:2 diet is, other than the need to stick to 500 or 600 calories for two days a week, there are no hard and fast rules. As with any new healthy habit though, it can take a bit of getting used to and you may find it challenging to start with as your body adjusts.

Choose your fasting days

The first thing you need to do is to decide which days will work best for you as fasting days. This might change from week to week to fit in with your social life or other plans but, generally speaking, most people find it easier to stick to the diet if they fast for the same two days every week. Also, for obvious reasons, many people opt not to fast on weekend days.

Whether you decide two consecutive days fasting or decide to have a gap between them is also up to you. Most people find it easier in terms of managing hunger and sticking to the diet to have their fasting days spread out of over the week but, if two days together suits you and you feel energetic and motivated, then that's fine.

When should I eat?

The second thing to decide is how you will consume your 500 or 600 calories on a fasting day. Again, this will be what works best for you and you will discover what suits you over time.

Many people opt for two meals: breakfast of around 100 calories, an evening meal of around 300 calories, leaving another 100 calories or so for a snack. Others find that they are happier if they don't eat anything at all until lunch. Some opt for saving all their calories for one reasonable-sized meal a day, either at lunchtime or in the evening, while – at the other end of the spectrum – some find it works for them to graze their way through fasting days, eating three mini meals spaced throughout the day.

What to eat

You can, of course, eat anything you like in theory, so long as you don't exceed your calorie quota. However, a fasting day is a great day to boost your health as well as your waistline by focusing on fruit and veg as they are bulky, so fill you up, and are low in calories.

Aim to include lean protein in low-calorie form; protein makes you feel full and you are more likely to preserve muscle tissue while restricting calories if you do. Good choices are prawns, tofu, tuna canned in water, grilled fish, chicken breast and eggs.

You won't be able to eat large carbohydrate portions on fasting days as they are relatively high in calories but make sure what you do choose is as unprocessed and high in fibre as possible; opt for wholemeal bread, wholewheat pasta, wholegrain cereals and so on.

Keeping a diary

To find a pattern of food intake that allows you to stick to the 5:2 diet, try keeping a food and mood diary. Jotting down what you eat and when and any accompanying feelings – for example, of hunger, wavering willpower or feeling motivated – can help you to tailor future fasting days to make them easier for you.

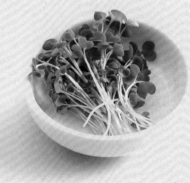

5 top tips to make
5:2 work for you

1 Be flexible: be prepared to test different fasting day routines until you find the one that works best for you.

2 Keep out of temptation's way: fasting days are surprisingly doable with a positive mindset and some forward planning but there's no point in testing your willpower if you can avoid it, so hide the biscuit tin and steer clear of the confectionary aisle of your supermarket on fasting days.

3 Find a fasting buddy: research shows that people dieting with friends to support them manage better so encourage a partner or friend to join you.

4 Keep busy: part of planning a successful fasting day is thinking about how you will occupy yourself so you are focusing on things other than food.

5 Stay positive: just about everyone trying to lose weight has frustrating periods when the weight won't come off or times when they fall off the diet wagon. Don't beat yourself up about it and don't give up. Try to focus on the weight you've already lost and consider every week that you stick with your fasting days as worth patting yourself on the back for.

Coping with hunger

There's no denying that 500 or 600 calories isn't a lot and some may find the 5:2 diet tricky at first but most long-term fans of the diet say that they are not unduly troubled by hunger pangs after a few weeks.

Dealing with initial hunger pangs can be as simple as realizing that nothing dreadful is going to happen if you feel hungry for a day. We are so used to eating whenever we feel the slightest hunger that this can feel strange at first, but you can learn to appreciate the physical feeling of hunger you get on a fasting day as you know that you are in tune with your body and are learning to be able to savour food without overloading your system.

Be aware that hunger pangs often come in waves; although you may be hungry now, you probably won't be in 20 minutes if you focus on something else. Simple activities such as phoning a friend, hanging up the washing or going for a walk will distract you from hunger.

Fluid is your friend

Stay hydrated is important at all times but especially on fasting days. Water drunk on its own will temporarily take the edge off a hunger pang and incorporated into food, such as soup, will increase satiety (the feeling of fullness that food gives).

You don't need to stick to plain water, though. Black tea and coffee, herbal teas and calorie-free beverages all count towards your fluid intake too.

Alcohol, on the other hand, is one of the least sensible choices. At around 100 calories for a small glass of wine, it will use up your calorie allocation and can also stimulate the appetite, so aim to make fasting days alcohol-free days too.

Don't guess

It's important, especially in the first few weeks, to accurately weigh or measure out everything you eat. You are almost certainly going to be wrong if you try estimating how much a portion of cereal or an apple, for example, weigh, which could add 'hidden' calories, jeopardizing your weight loss and diluting the health benefits.

It is also important to accurately measure the ingredients for the recipes in this book, so that they don't exceed the calorie counts given.

So, before you embark on your first fasting day, make sure you've got kitchen scales and a measuring jug, both of which are available quite cheaply.

What about exercise?

An exercise programme will certainly complement your 5:2 diet and will bring with it many health benefits, including stronger bones and a healthy heart.

There's no reason you shouldn't work out on your fasting days and, in fact, the latest evidence suggests that exercising while you are fasting means that the body has to use fat as its primary fuel which is great news when it comes to getting rid of unwanted bulges.

However, if you're completely new to exercise, it's probably best to ease yourself in by exercising on non-fasting days only to begin with. Listen to your body and always stop exercising immediately if you feel faint or light-headed.

Non-fasting days

The great appeal of the 5:2 diet is that for most of the week you don't have to think about calories at all!

Research has shown that, contrary to what you might expect, intermittent fasters are very unlikely to go on a binge on their non-fasting days. Instead, 5:2 eating appears to help to naturally regulate your appetite over time, making you more aware of food so that you enjoy only as much as you need on non-fasting days.

You can pretty much eat as you like, as long as you don't overdo it, and there's lots of scope for treats, but non-fasting days should include a good balance of wholesome food too.

So aim to include five portions of a wide variety of fruit and vegetables a day (as you should do on fasting days too). You should also try to eat minimally processed carbohydrates and some protein each day (each should ideally take up a quarter of the space on your plate at a meal).

Including dairy foods or fortified alternatives, such as soya, rice or nut milks, daily will ensure that you have enough calcium in your diet.

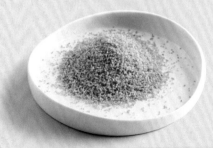

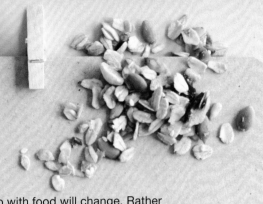

You and food

With time, your relationship with food will change. Rather than food being your master, as is often the case with those who have struggled with their weight over the years, you are likely to start to feel in control of food once more. Many people who adopt 5:2 eating as a way of life say that it is very empowering, once they've cracked fasting days.

This is because 5:2 eating can help you to be more in tune with your body, particularly your appetite and hunger cues. The boost in confidence that this gives is an important step in developing a healthier relationship with food. For some people, this feeling of empowerment in more marked than for others but, for all of us, feeling more in control of what we eat is to be welcomed.

Using this book

The 100 delicious recipes in this book offer calorie-controlled options for breakfast, snacks, lunch, dinner and even desserts. Packed with flavour and variety, they're aimed at filling you up the healthy, low-calorie way, making following the 5:2 diet easy. Included in the recipes are some special treats that you will find satisfying for both fasting and non-fasting days alike.

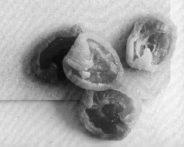

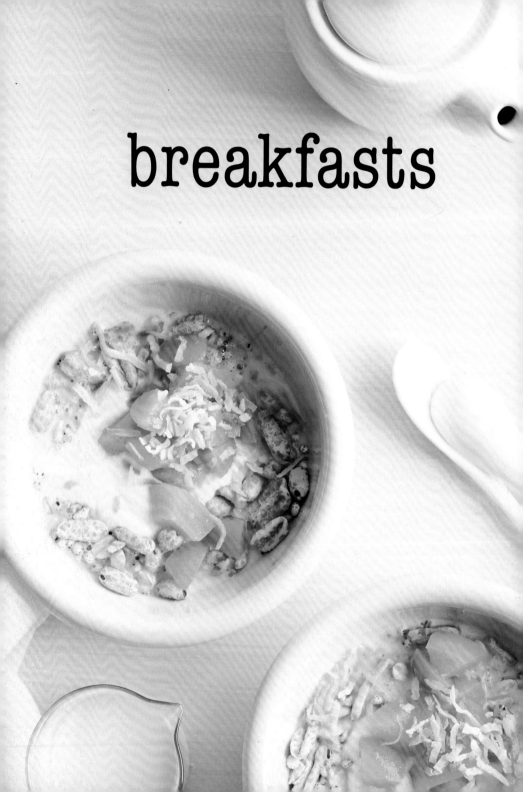

breakfasts

apricot & coconut muesli

serves 6
prep time 15 minutes
nutritional count per serving 3g total fat (1.5g saturated fat);
585kJ (140 cal); 19.9g carbohydrate; 6.9g protein; 2.7g fibre

140
calorie count per serving

90g (3oz) rolled oats
10g (⅓oz) puffed millet
10g (⅓oz) puffed whole wheat
160ml (5½fl oz) skimmed milk
2 tablespoons fat-free natural yogurt
135g (5oz) canned apricots in natural juice, drained and diced
3 teaspoons shredded coconut, toasted

1 For the muesli mixture, combine oats, millet and
wheat in a small bowl.
2 Place 18g (½oz) muesli in each bowl; top with milk,
yogurt, apricots and coconut. Store remaining
muesli in an airtight container and use for
breakfast on another day.

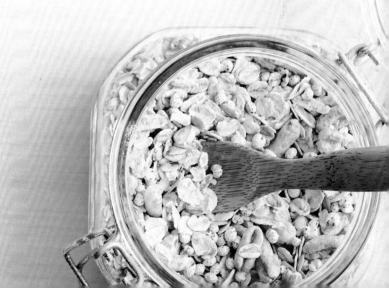

rice flake porridge with banana

serves 2
prep + cook time 20 minutes (+ standing)
nutritional count per serving 0.7g total fat
(0.1g saturated fat); 614kJ (147 cal); 33g
carbohydrate; 1.9g protein; 1.5g fibre

25g (1oz) rice flakes
180ml (6⅓fl oz) water
60ml (2fl oz) rice milk
1 small banana (130g), sliced thinly
pinch ground cinnamon
1 tablespoon honey

1 Combine rice flakes and the
water in a small bowl, cover; stand
overnight.
2 Place undrained rice mixture in
medium saucepan; bring to the
boil, stirring. Reduce heat; simmer,
uncovered, stirring occasionally,
about 5 minutes or until porridge is
thick and creamy.
3 Divide porridge and milk between
bowls; top with banana, cinnamon
and honey.

tip Rice flakes are available at health-
food shops and online.

147
calorie count per serving

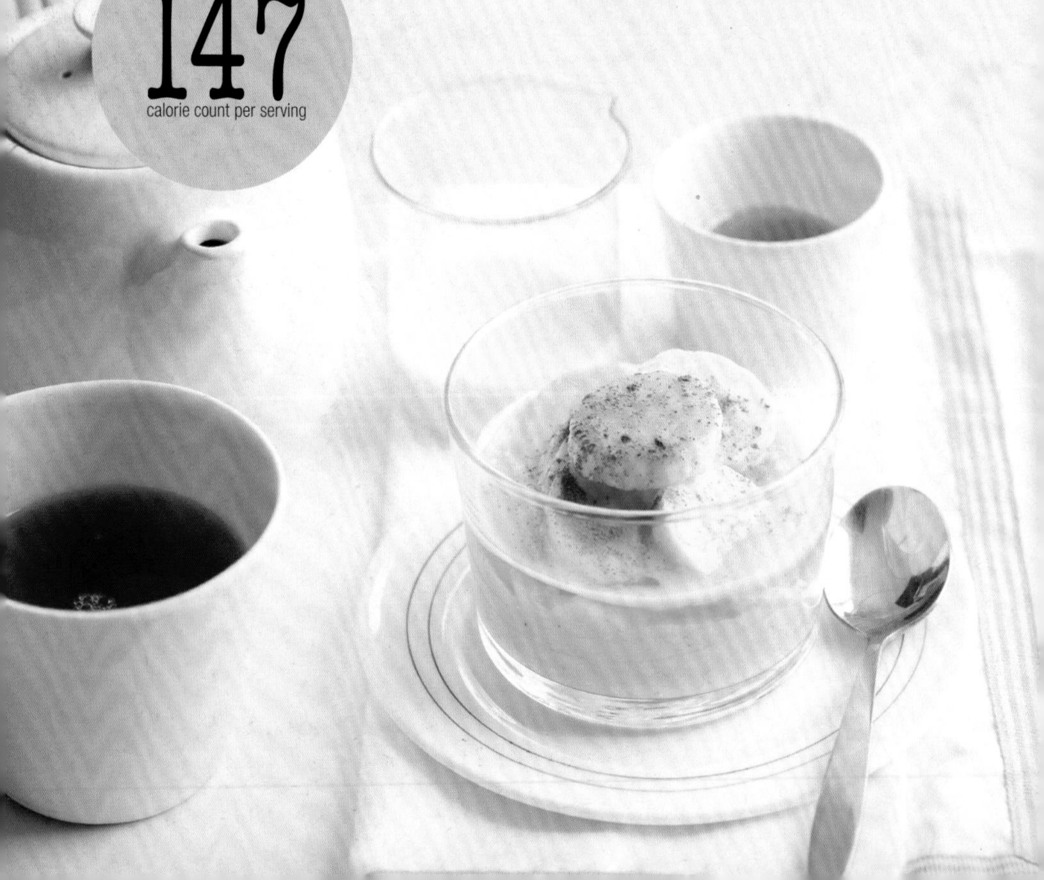

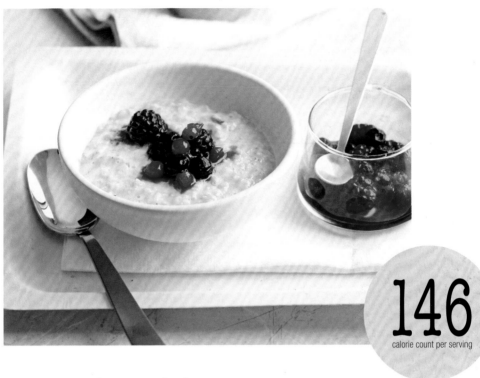

146
calorie count per serving

oat porridge with berry compote

serves 2
prep time 15 minutes
nutritional count per serving 2.1g total fat
(0.4g saturated fat); 610kJ (146 cal); 26.3g
carbohydrate; 6.1g protein; 3.8g fibre

150g (5oz) frozen mixed berries
1 tablespoon caster sugar
2 tablespoons boiling water
45g (1½oz) rolled oats
125ml (4fl oz) skimmed milk
125ml (4fl oz) boiling water, extra

1 Place berries in a small heatproof
bowl, add sugar and the boiling
water; stir until sugar dissolves.
2 Combine oats, milk and the extra
boiling water in medium saucepan;
cook, stirring, about 5 minutes or
until porridge comes to the boil and
thickens (it should coat the back of
a spoon). Remove from heat, cover;
stand about 5 minutes or until thick
and creamy.
3 Drain berries just before serving.
Serve porridge topped with berries.

tip If porridge becomes too thick,
stir in a little extra boiling water.

banana, mango & raspberry smoothie

serves 2
prep time 10 minutes
nutritional count per serving 0.5g total fat
(0.1g saturated fat); 644kJ (154 cal); 29g
carbohydrate; 6.7g protein; 3.9g fibre

1 small banana (130g), chopped coarsely
1 small mango (300g), chopped coarsely
50g (2oz) frozen raspberries
250ml (8fl oz) skimmed milk

1 Blend ingredients until smooth.

tip For a super-chilled summery
smoothie, freeze the chopped banana
and the mango overnight before using.

154
calorie count per serving

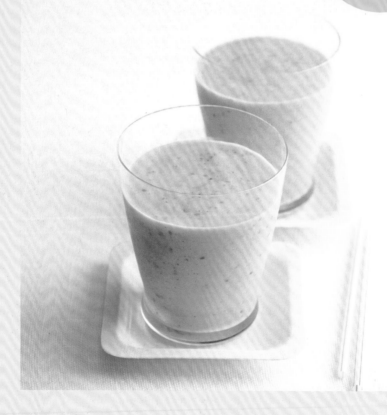

blueberry & apple bircher muesli

serves 2
prep time 15 minutes (+ refrigeration)
nutritional count per serving 2.1g total fat
(0.4g saturated fat); 635kJ (152 cal); 26.7g
carbohydrate; 5.1g protein; 3.5g fibre

45g (1½oz) rolled oats
125ml (4fl oz) skimmed milk
60ml (2fl oz) unsweetened apple juice
35g (1½oz) fresh blueberries
1 small green apple (130g), unpeeled,
    cored, sliced thinly

1 Combine oats, milk and juice in
small bowl, cover; refrigerate 3 hours
or overnight.
2 Serve muesli topped with berries
and apple.

tip For a different option, grate the
apple coarsely.

152
calorie count per serving

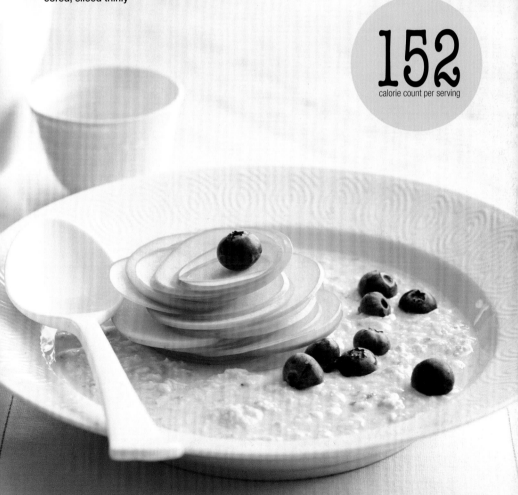

crêpes with banana & passionfruit syrup

serves 2
prep + cook time 20 minutes
nutritional count per serving 0.3g total fat
(0g saturated fat); 594kJ (142 cal); 28.8g
carbohydrate; 3.6g protein; 4.4g fibre

35g (1½oz) plain flour
1 tablespoon skimmed milk
80ml (3fl oz) water
2 teaspoons honey
2 tablespoons passionfruit pulp
1 small banana (130g), sliced thickly

142
calorie count per serving

1 Sift flour into small bowl; gradually whisk in combined milk and the water until batter is smooth. Heat medium non-stick frying pan over medium heat; pour in half the batter, tilt pan to cover base with batter. Cook crêpe until browned lightly, loosening edge with spatula. Turn crêpe; brown the other side. Remove crêpe from pan; cover to keep warm. Repeat with remaining batter.
2 Meanwhile, combine honey and pulp in a small microwave-safe jug; microwave on MEDIUM (50%) about 30 seconds or until hot.
3 Serve crêpes with banana and hot passionfruit syrup.

tip You need about two passionfruits.

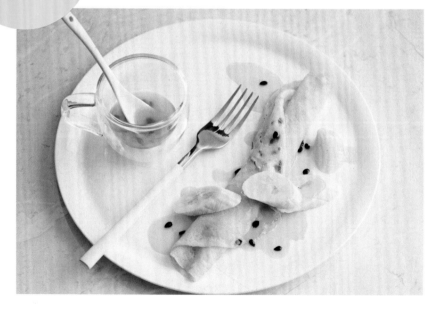

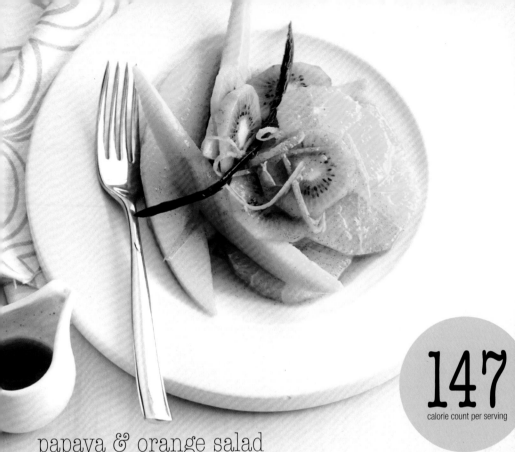

147
calorie count per serving

papaya & orange salad

serves 2
prep + cook time 20 minutes (+ refrigeration)
nutritional count per serving 0.3g total fat
(0g saturated fat); 614kJ (147 cal); 29.9g
carbohydrate; 2.9g protein; 6.5g fibre

3 small oranges (540g)
80ml (3fl oz) water
1 tablespoon grated palm sugar
1 vanilla pod, split lengthways
¼ small papaya (165g), peeled, sliced
    thickly
1 medium kiwi fruit (85g), peeled, sliced
    thinly

1 Using one orange only, peel thinly,
then slice rind finely (you need 1
tablespoon rind); squeeze and reserve
the juice (you need 80ml/3fl oz).
2 Combine reserved juice, the
water, sugar and vanilla pod in small
saucepan; bring to the boil. Reduce
heat; simmer, uncovered, about
5 minutes or until syrup thickens.
Remove from heat; stir in orange rind.
Refrigerate about 20 minutes or until
cool. Discard vanilla pod.
3 Peel and thinly slice remaining
oranges. Combine papaya, orange
and kiwi fruit in serving bowls; drizzle
with syrup, stand 10 minutes before
serving.

cherry parfait

serves 2
prep + cook time 20 minutes
nutritional count per serving 1g total fat
(0.2g saturated fat); 644kJ (154 cal); 27.3g
carbohydrate; 7.2g protein; 2g fibre

1 tablespoon caster sugar
2 tablespoons water
150g (5oz) fresh or frozen pitted cherries,
   halved
190g (7oz) fat-free natural yogurt
2 teaspoons vanilla extract
pinch ground cinnamon
2 tablespoons rolled oats, toasted

1 Combine the sugar, water and
cherries in medium saucepan; bring
to the boil. Reduce heat; simmer,
uncovered, for about 2 minutes or
until syrup thickens. Cool.
2 Meanwhile, combine yogurt, vanilla
and cinnamon in small bowl.
3 Divide half the cherry mixture
between two 180ml (6½fl oz) glasses.
Top with half the yogurt, then
remaining cherry mixture and yogurt.
Sprinkle with oats just before serving.

tips To toast the oats, stir them in a
heated small frying pan over medium
heat until browned lightly; or roast
them in the oven, on an oven tray.
Store the oats in a snap-lock bag and
sprinkle over the parfaits just before
serving. Parfaits can be made the
night before and kept, covered, in
the refrigerator.

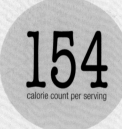

154
calorie count per serving

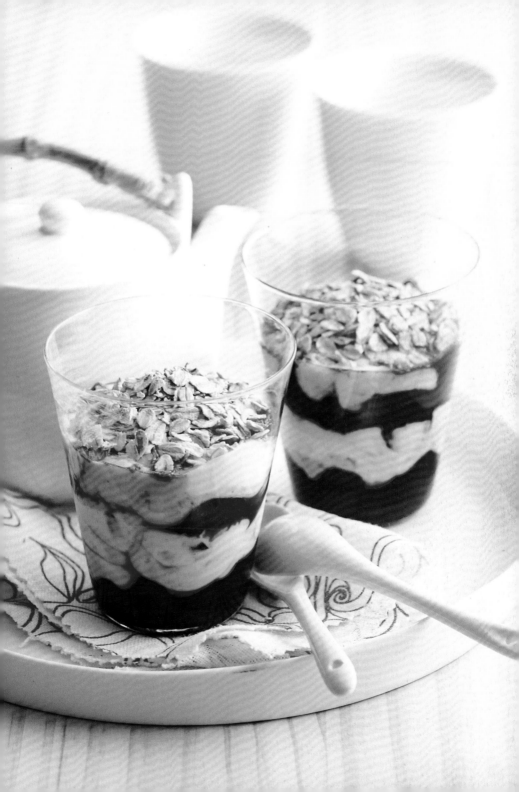

english muffin with mint & pineapple juice

serves 2
prep time 10 minutes
nutritional count per serving 0.7g total fat
(0.1g saturated fat); 631kJ (151 cal); 32g
carbohydrate; 6.2g protein; 7.1g fibre

300g (10oz) piece fresh peeled pineapple,
   chopped coarsely
2 small oranges (360g), peeled, quartered
12 fresh mint leaves
2 tablespoons lime juice
80ml (3fl oz) iced water
2 teaspoons jam or marmalade
1 wholemeal english muffin, split, toasted

1 Push pineapple, orange and mint
through juice extractor into medium
jug. Stir in lime juice and the water.
2 Spread jam on muffin; serve with
the juice.

tip For a super-chilled summery
smoothie, freeze the chopped
banana and the mango overnight
before using.

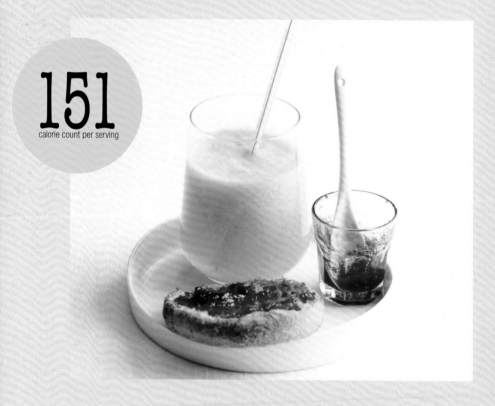

151
calorie count per serving

english muffin with beetroot juice

serves 2
prep time 10 minutes
nutritional count per serving 2.7g total fat
(1g saturated fat); 731kJ (172 cal); 26.2g
carbohydrate; 7.8g protein; 6.5g fibre

2 fresh small beetroot (200g), peeled,
   chopped coarsely
2 small apples (260g), unpeeled, chopped
   coarsely
40g (1½oz) baby spinach leaves
3cm (1¼-inch) piece fresh ginger (15g)
250ml (8fl oz) iced water
1 tablespoon ricotta
1 wholemeal english muffin (65g), split,
   toasted

1 Push beetroot, apple, spinach and
ginger through juice extractor into
medium jug. Stir in the water.
2 Spread cheese on muffin; serve
with juice.

tip If you prefer to drink chilled
juices, keep the vegetables and fruit
refrigerated before juicing; or serve
the juice over crushed ice.

172
calorie count per serving

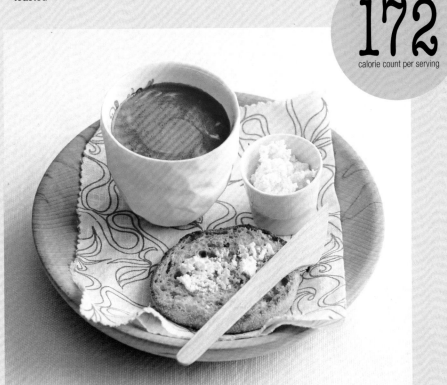

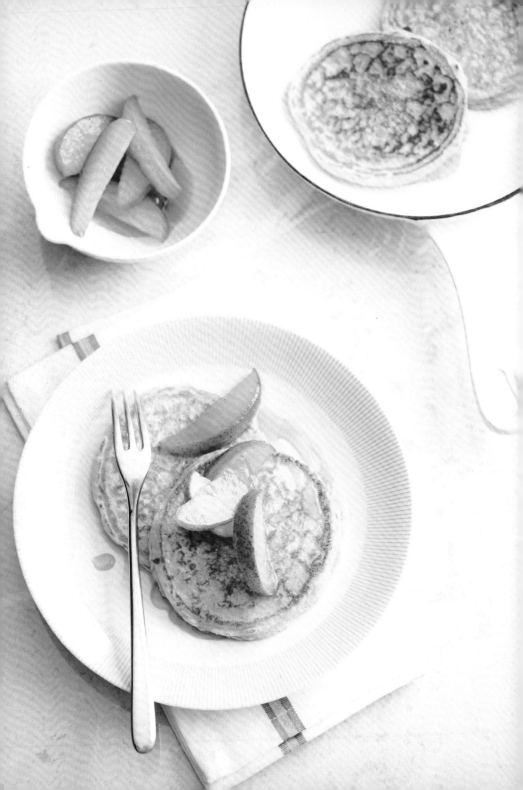

pancakes with honey pears

serves 2
prep + cook time 25 minutes
nutritional count per serving 0.4g total fat
(0.1g saturated fat); 627kJ (150 cal); 40.7g
carbohydrate; 6g protein; 2.2g fibre

1 small pear (180g), unpeeled, cored,
  cut into wedges
1 tablespoon honey
180ml (6⅓fl oz) water
2 teaspoons lemon juice
50g (2oz) self-raising flour
¼ teaspoon ground cinnamon
80ml (3fl oz) skimmed milk
1 egg white

1 Combine the pear, honey, water
and juice in medium frying pan; bring
to the boil. Reduce heat; simmer,
covered, about 5 minutes or until
pears start to soften. Uncover;
simmer, about 5 minutes or until
pears are tender and syrup is thick.

2 Meanwhile, sift flour and cinnamon
into medium bowl; gradually whisk in
milk until batter is smooth. Beat egg
white in small bowl with electric mixer
until soft peaks form. Fold egg white
into batter.

3 Heat large non-stick frying pan
over medium heat; pour 60ml
(2fl oz) batter for each pancake into
pan (you can cook two at a time).
Cook pancakes until bubbles appear
on the surface; turn and cook until
the other side is browned. Remove
from pan; cover to keep warm.
Repeat with remaining batter to make
a total of four pancakes.

4 Serve pancakes topped with pears
and syrup.

grilled vegetables with ricotta

serves 2
prep + cook time 30 minutes
nutritional count per serving 4g total fat
(1.1g saturated fat); 742kJ (177 cal); 24.5g
carbohydrate; 8.2g protein; 4.4g fibre

1 medium courgette (120g), sliced thinly
  lengthways
1 medium yellow pepper (200g), sliced
  thickly
1 medium tomato (150g), halved
2 slices ciabatta bread (70g)
cooking oil spray
1 tablespoon ricotta
1 tablespoon small fresh basil leaves
30g (1oz) rocket leaves

1 Spray courgette, pepper, tomato
and bread with a little cooking oil;
season vegetables. Cook vegetables
and bread, in batches, on heated
griddle pan (or grill) until vegetables
are tender and bread is browned
lightly on both sides.
2 Spread cheese onto toasted
bread; sprinkle with basil. Serve with
vegetables and rocket.

tips The vegetables can be cooked
the night before; store them, covered,
in the refrigerator. Toast the bread just
before serving.

177
calorie count per serving

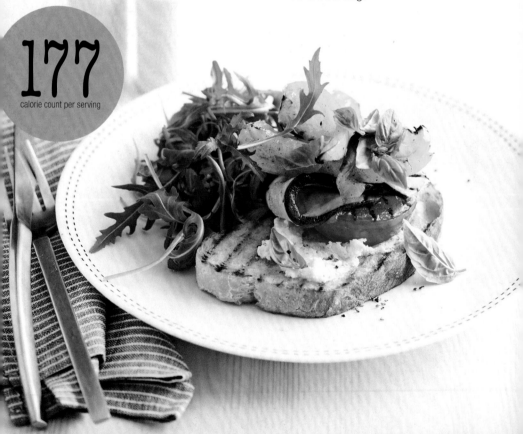

rye toasts with roasted tomato & basil

serves 2
prep + cook time 15 minutes
nutritional count per serving 2.1g total fat
(0.6g saturated fat); 640kJ (153 cal); 20.2g
carbohydrate; 10.6g protein; 3.9g fibre

2 small tomatoes (180g), each cut into
  6 wedges
1 tablespoon balsamic vinegar
2 slices prosciutto (30g)
2 tablespoons low-fat cottage cheese
2 slices rye bread (90g), toasted
2 tablespoons basil leaves

1 Preheat oven to 220°C.
2 Combine tomato and vinegar in
small shallow baking dish. Place
prosciutto on oven tray. Roast,
uncovered, about 10 minutes or
until tomato softens and prosciutto
is crisp.
3 Spread cheese over toast; top
with tomato, prosciutto and basil.
Season to taste.

153
calorie count per serving

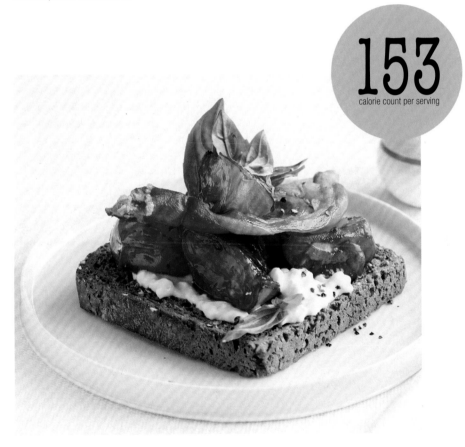

vegetable rösti with ham & roasted tomatoes

serves 2
prep + cook time 30 minutes
nutritional count per serving 2.2g total fat
(0.6g saturated fat); 627kJ (150 cal); 17.6g
carbohydrate; 11.7g protein; 6.3g fibre

60g (2oz) wafer-thin reduced-fat ham
125g (4oz) cherry tomatoes
1 small potato (150g), unpeeled, grated
  coarsely
1 medium fresh beetroot (175g), peeled,
  grated coarsely
1 medium courgette (120g), grated
  coarsely
1 egg white, beaten lightly
40g (1½oz) baby spinach leaves

1 Preheat oven to 220°C. Line oven
tray with baking parchment.
2 Place ham and tomatoes on
tray; roast about 10 minutes or until
tomatoes start to collapse.
3 To make rösti, combine the potato,
beetroot, courgette and egg white in
a large bowl; season. Divide mixture
into four portions. Cook one portion
in a heated large non-stick frying pan
over medium heat, pressing down
firmly to flatten, until browned both
sides and cooked through. Remove
from pan, place on oven tray; transfer
to oven to keep warm. Repeat with
remaining vegetable mixture.
4 Combine warm tomatoes with
spinach in medium bowl. Serve
spinach mixture with ham and rösti.

150
calorie count per serving

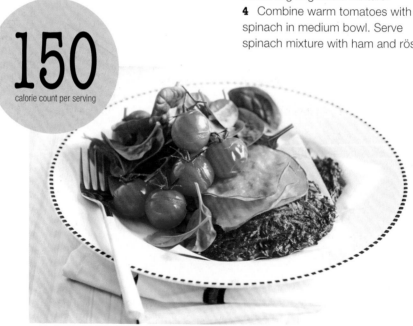

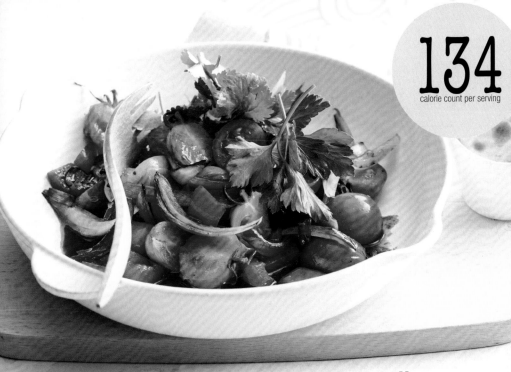

chunky mexican-style salsa with tortillas

serves 2
prep + cook time 25 minutes
nutritional count per serving 1.1g total fat
(0.1g saturated fat); 560kJ (134 cal); 21.5g
carbohydrate; 5.8g protein; 5.8g fibre

1 small red onion (100g), cut into thin
  wedges
pinch dried chilli flakes
400g (13oz) mixed baby tomatoes, halved
1 medium red pepper (200g), chopped
  coarsely
2 tablespoons water
1 tablespoon balsamic vinegar
2 small white tortillas (56g)
2 tablespoons fresh coriander leaves
2 tablespoons fresh flat-leaf parsley leaves

1 Heat lightly oiled non-stick frying
pan over medium heat; cook onion
and chilli, stirring, until onion softens.
Add tomato, pepper, the water and
vinegar; bring to the boil. Reduce
heat; simmer, uncovered, stirring
occasionally, about 15 minutes or
until pepper is tender and tomato
begins to soften. Season to taste.
2 Meanwhile, cook tortillas, one at
a time, in heated small frying pan
about 1 minute on each side or until
browned lightly and warmed through.
3 Serve tomato mixture with tortillas;
sprinkle with coriander and parsley.

tips You can warm the tortillas in the
microwave; follow the instructions on
the packet. Omit the chilli if you like.

mixed mushroom & herb omelette

serves 2
prep + cook time 20 minutes
nutritional count per serving 3.1g total fat
(0.8g saturated fat); 523kJ (125 cal); 3g
carbohydrate; 18.2g protein; 6.5g fibre

5 button mushrooms (60g), sliced thickly
1 flat mushroom (80g), sliced thinly
150g (5oz) oyster mushrooms, sliced
    thickly
60g (2oz) baby spinach leaves
1 egg
5 egg whites
2 tablespoons water
3 spring onions, sliced thinly
3 tablespoons finely chopped fresh
    flat-leaf parsley

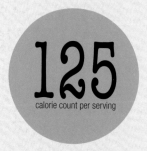

125
calorie count per serving

1 Heat lightly oiled medium non-
stick frying pan over medium heat;
cook mushrooms, stirring, about
5 minutes or until browned lightly and
tender. Transfer to medium bowl, stir
in spinach; season to taste. Cover to
keep warm.

2 Meanwhile, whisk egg and egg
whites in medium jug until combined
and frothy; whisk in the water, half the
onion and half the parsley.

3 Pour half the egg mixture into
same heated pan; tilt pan to cover
base with egg mixture. Cook omelette
over medium heat until almost set.
Spoon half the mushrooms over
half the omelette. Use a spatula to
fold the omelette over mushrooms.
Carefully slide omelette onto plate;
cover with foil to keep warm.
Repeat with remaining egg mixture
and mushrooms to make another
omelette.

4 Serve omelette immediately
sprinkled with remaining onion and
parsley.

tip We used oyster mushrooms for
their unique flavour, but you can use
any combination of mushrooms you
like, to collectively weigh about 300g
(10oz).

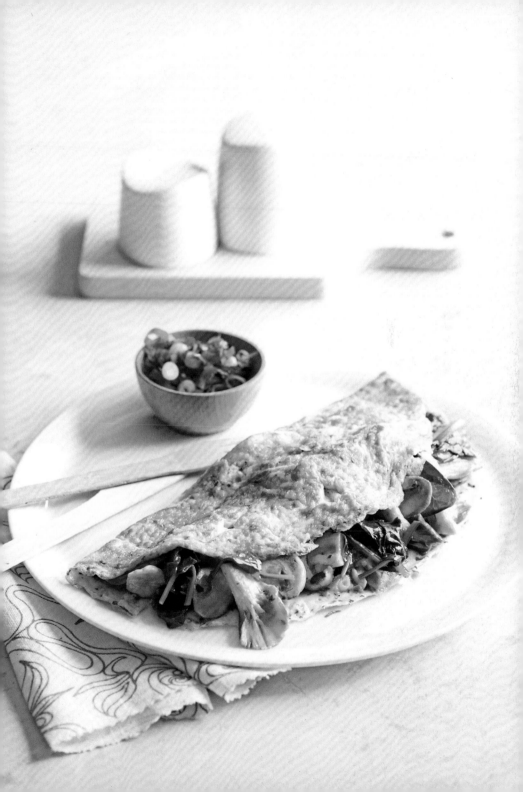

snacks

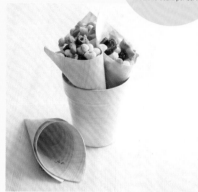

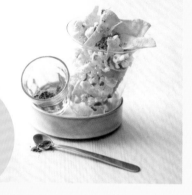

spiced popcorn

serves 2
prep + cook time 10 minutes
nutritional count per serving 1.1g total
fat (0.3g saturated fat); 184kJ (44 cal); 5.5g
carbohydrate; 2g protein; 1.8g fibre

1 tablespoon popping corn
½ teaspoon ground coriander
½ teaspoon ground cumin
¼ teaspoon ground cinnamon
15g (½oz) mini plain pappadoms

1 Place popping corn in a paper
bag; secure loosely with kitchen
string. Microwave bag on MEDIUM-
HIGH (75%) about 4 minutes or until
popped. Carefully remove bag from
microwave with tongs; stand
2 minutes before opening.
2 Meanwhile, dry-fry coriander,
cumin and cinnamon in heated small
frying pan until fragrant.
3 Break pappadoms into pieces
into medium bowl; add popcorn and
spices, toss gently to combine.

fruit nibble mix

serves 8
prep time 10 minutes
nutritional count per serving 0.1g total
fat (0g saturated fat); 217kJ (52 cal); 11.7g
carbohydrate; 0.7g protein; 1.4g fibre

3 rosemary and sea salt grissini
30g (1oz) puffed corn
38g (1⅓oz) dried apricots, quartered
38g (1⅓oz) dried pears, coarsely chopped
42g (1½oz) pitted dried dates, coarsely
    chopped

1 Break grissini into small pieces
into a medium bowl; add puffed corn,
apricots, pears and dates; mix well.

tip Grissini are crisp, thin
breadsticks; use any flavour you like.

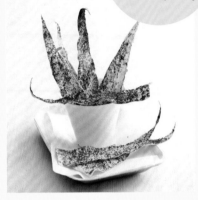

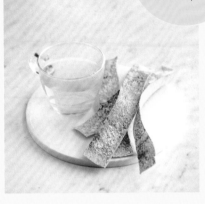

seeded mustard crisps

serves 2
prep + cook time 20 minutes
nutritional count per serving 1.2g total fat (0.2g saturated fat); 201kJ (48 cal); 6.6g carbohydrate; 1.5g protein; 0.9g fibre

1 thin wholemeal wrap
cooking oil spray
2 teaspoons dijon mustard
1 teaspoon poppy seeds
½ teaspoon sweet paprika
¼ teaspoon sea salt flakes

1 Preheat oven to 180°C. Line oven tray with baking parchment.
2 Spray wrap with cooking oil; spread with mustard, then sprinkle with poppy seeds, paprika and sea salt flakes. Cut wrap in half crossways; cut each half into long thin triangles.
3 Place triangles on tray; bake about 4 minutes or until crisp. Cool on trays.

cinnamon crisps

serves 2
prep + cook time 10 minutes
nutritional count per serving 0.8g total fat (0.1g saturated fat); 230kJ (55 cal); 10.4g carbohydrate; 1.4g protein; 0.6g fibre

1 thin wholemeal wrap
cooking oil spray
2 teaspoons icing sugar
¼ teaspoon ground cinnamon

1 Preheat oven to 180°C. Line an oven tray with baking parchment.
2 Spray wrap with cooking oil. Sift sugar and cinnamon over wrap.
3 Cut wrap in half crossways; cut each half into wide strips. Place on oven tray; bake about 4 minutes or until crisp. Cool on trays.

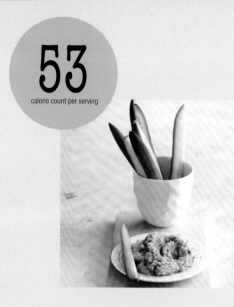

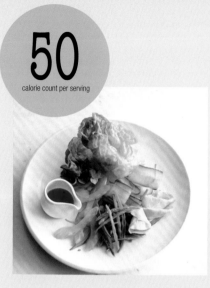

chickpea & cumin dip

serves 2
prep time 15 minutes
nutritional count per serving 1g total fat
(0.1g saturated fat); 222kJ (53 cal); 7.3g
carbohydrate; 3g protein; 2.9g fibre

125g (4oz) canned chickpeas, rinsed
   and drained
1 tablespoon lemon juice
1 garlic clove, crushed
¼ teaspoon ground cumin
½ cucumber (130g)

1 Blend or process chickpeas,
lemon juice, garlic clove and cumin
until smooth.
2 Sprinkle dip with a pinch of ground
cumin; serve with cucumber, cut into
wedges.

ham salad lettuce wraps

serves 2
prep time 15 minutes
nutritional count per serving 1g total fat
(0.2g saturated fat); 209kJ (50 cal); 4.9g
carbohydrate; 4.2g protein; 2.5g fibre

½ cucumber (130g)
1 celery stalk (150g)
45g (1½oz) thinly sliced mangetout
30g (1oz) wafer thin reduced-fat ham
6 butter lettuce leaves
1 tablespoon sweet chilli sauce

1 Slice cucumber into ribbons. Thinly
slice celery on the diagonal.
2 Divide cucumber, celery, sliced
mangetout and ham between lettuce
leaves.
3 Drizzle with sweet chilli sauce.

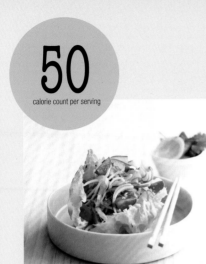

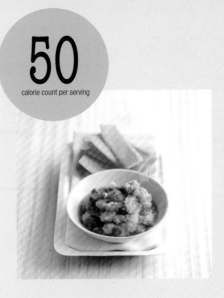

50 calorie count per serving

50 calorie count per serving

thai salad cups

serves 2
prep time 20 minutes
nutritional count per serving 0.9g total
fat (0.1g saturated fat); 209kJ (50 cal); 6.2g
carbohydrate; 2.6g protein; 3.4g fibre

2 tablespoons lemon juice
¼ teaspoon sesame oil
1 teaspoon fish sauce
125g (4oz) cherry tomatoes, quartered
40g (1½oz) bean sprouts
½ cucumber (130g), sliced into ribbons
1 small red onion (100g), sliced thinly
6 tablespoons coarsely chopped fresh
   coriander
50g (2oz) finely shredded iceberg lettuce
2 small iceberg lettuce leaves

1 To make sesame dressing, combine
juice, oil and sauce in small bowl.
2 Combine tomato, sprouts,
cucumber, onion, coriander and
shredded lettuce in medium bowl.
Add dressing; toss gently to combine.
3 Spoon salad into lettuce leaves to
serve.

garlicky aubergine dip

serves 2
prep + cook time 35 minutes
nutritional count per serving 0.5g total
fat (0g saturated fat); 209kJ (50cal); 6.7g
carbohydrate; 2g protein; 4.5g fibre

1 small aubergine (230g), halved
1 clove garlic, chopped coarsely
2 tablespoons lemon juice
1 spring onion, sliced thinly
1 medium carrot (120g), sliced thinly

1 Preheat oven to 200°C. Line oven
tray with baking parchment.
2 Place aubergine on oven tray;
bake about 25 minutes or until soft.
Cool; remove skin, then blend or
process aubergine with garlic and
juice until almost smooth. Stir half the
onion into the dip; season to taste.
3 Serve dip sprinkled with remaining
onion; serve with carrot.

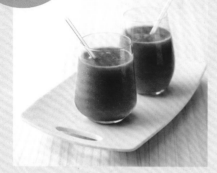

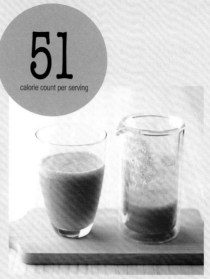

melon & raspberry frappé

serves 2
prep time 10 minutes
nutritional count per serving 0.5g total fat
(0g saturated fat); 138kJ (33 cal); 9.6g
carbohydrate; 1.1g protein; 3.6g fibre

400g (13oz) watermelon, deseeded, peeled
   and coarsely chopped
100g (3½oz) frozen raspberries
1 teaspoon finely grated lime rind
1½ tablespoons lime juice
12 ice cubes

1   Place all the ingredients in a
blender and blend until mixture is
smooth.

pineapple & strawberry lassi

serves 2
prep time 10 minutes
nutritional count per serving 0.2g total fat
(0.1g saturated fat); 213kJ (51 cal); 8.2g
carbohydrate; 4.9g protein; 1.9g fibre

125ml (4fl oz) skimmed milk
2 tablespoons low-fat natural yogurt
100g (3½oz) fresh pineapple, peeled and
   coarsely chopped
125g (4oz) strawberries, halved
12 ice cubes

1   Place all the ingredients in a
blender and blend until smooth.

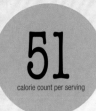

51
calorie count per serving

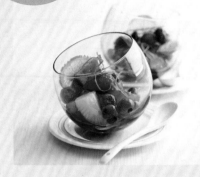

48
calorie count per serving

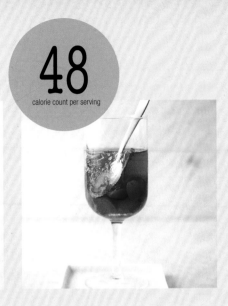

berry & lime
fruit salad

serves 2
prep time 10 minutes
nutritional count per serving 0.2g total fat (0g saturated fat); 213kJ (51 cal); 9.1g carbohydrate; 1.5g protein; 2.3g fibre

125g (4oz) strawberries, quartered
75g (3oz) blueberries
1 teaspoon finely grated lime rind
1 tablespoon lime juice
2 teaspoons icing sugar
1 tablespoon finely shredded fresh mint

1 Combine strawberries, blueberries, rind, juice, icing sugar and mint in a small bowl; stand for at least 10 minutes before serving.

raspberry &
grape jelly

serves 2
prep time 15 minutes (+ cooling & refrigeration)
nutritional count per serving 0.1g total fat (0g saturated fat); 201kJ (48 cal); 11.3g carbohydrate; 0.6g protein; 0.7g fibre

9g (½oz) sachet sugar-free raspberry-
  flavoured jelly crystals
430ml (15fl oz) boiling water
150g (5oz) seedless red grapes, halved

1 Combine jelly crystals in medium heatproof jug with boiling water, stirring until jelly dissolves; cool.
2 Divide grapes between two 250ml (8fl oz) glasses. Pour jelly mixture into glasses, cover; refrigerate 3 hours or overnight.

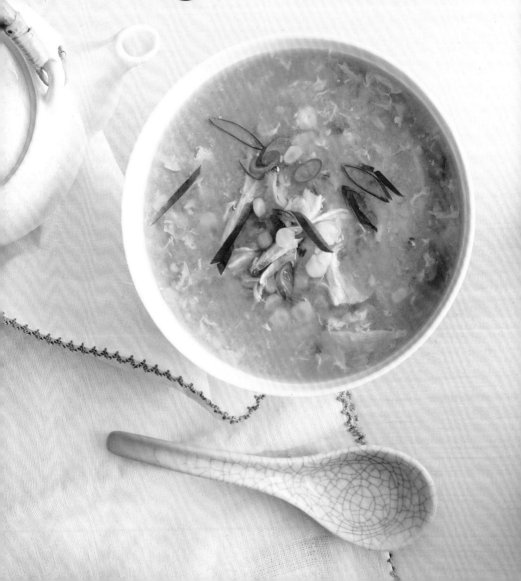

lunches &
light meals

chicken & corn soup

serves 2
prep + cook time 25 minutes
nutritional count per serving 5.6g total fat (1.6g saturated fat);
1513kJ (362 cal); 44g carbohydrate; 50.2g protein; 9g fibre

1 trimmed corn cob (250g), kernels removed
2cm (¾-inch) piece fresh ginger (10g), grated
1 garlic clove, crushed
2 spring onions, sliced thinly
250g (8oz) canned creamed corn
1 tablespoon japanese soy sauce
1 litre (1¾ pints) salt-reduced chicken stock
320g (11oz) skinless cooked chicken, chopped
1 egg white, beaten lightly

1 Heat large non-stick saucepan over medium heat; cook corn, ginger,
garlic and half the onion, stirring, until fragrant. Add creamed corn,
sauce and stock; bring to the boil.
2 Add chicken, reduce heat; simmer, uncovered, 10 minutes.
Gradually stir in egg white. Season to taste.
3 Serve soup sprinkled with remaining onion.

tip Reheat soup in a microwave on HIGH (100%)
for about 1½ minutes, stirring
halfway through heating.

362
calorie count per serving

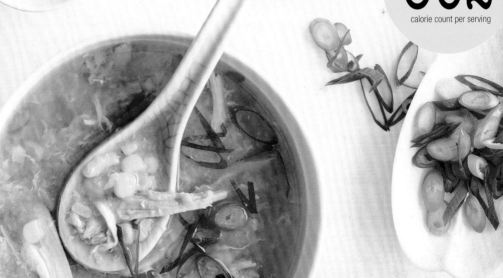

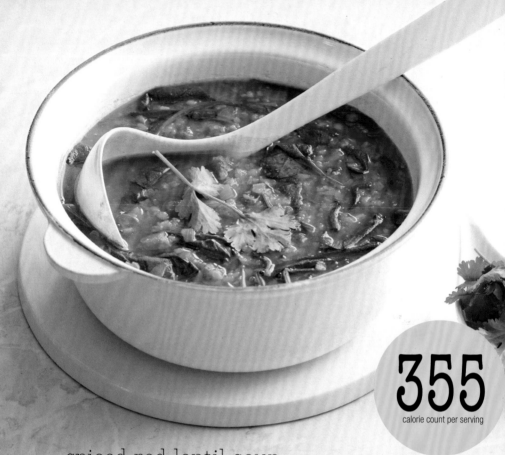

355 calorie count per serving

spiced red lentil soup

serves 2
prep + cook time 35 minutes
nutritional count per serving 7.9g total fat
(1.5g saturated fat); 1484kJ (355 cal); 35.7g
carbohydrate; 29.7g protein; 13.8g fibre

1 large brown onion (200g), chopped finely
1 fresh long red chilli, sliced thinly
1 tablespoon mild curry paste
500ml (17fl oz) chicken stock
500ml (17fl oz) water
400g (13oz) canned diced tomatoes
100g (3½oz) red lentils, rinsed
100g (3½oz) piece smoked ham, cut into
    1cm (½-inch) pieces
150g (5oz) baby spinach leaves
3 tablespoons fresh coriander leaves

1 Heat medium non-stick saucepan
over medium heat; cook onion and
chilli, stirring, until onion softens.
Add curry paste; cook, stirring, about
1 minute or until fragrant.
2 Add stock, the water, undrained
tomatoes and lentils; bring to the boil.
Reduce heat; simmer, covered, about
20 minutes or until lentils are tender.
Stir in ham and spinach; return to the
boil. Season to taste.
3 Serve soup topped with coriander.

tip Reheat the soup, covered, in a
microwave on HIGH (100%) for about
1½ minutes.

hot & sour vegetable soup

serves 2
prep + cook time 25 minutes
nutritional count per serving 5.4g total fat
(0.7g saturated fat); 1672kJ (400 cal); 59.4g
carbohydrate; 21.3g protein; 13.3g fibre

90g (3oz) dried soba noodles
1 tablespoon tom yum paste
2 kaffir lime leaves, crushed
1 fresh long red chilli, halved
500ml (17fl oz) water
500ml (17fl oz) chicken stock
1 large carrot (180g), cut into matchsticks
1 medium red pepper (200g), sliced thinly
100g (3½oz) button mushrooms, sliced
    thinly
175g (6oz) tenderstem broccoli, chopped
    coarsely
100g (3½oz) mangetout, sliced thinly
2 spring onions, sliced thinly
1½ tablespoons lime juice
1 tablespoon fish sauce
40g (1½oz) bean sprouts
1 tablespoon each fresh mint and
    coriander leaves

1 Cook noodles in large saucepan
of boiling water until tender; drain.
2 Heat large non-stick saucepan
over medium heat; cook paste, lime
leaves and chilli, stirring, until fragrant.
Add the water and stock; bring to the
boil, stirring.
3 Reduce heat; simmer, uncovered,
5 minutes. Add carrot, pepper,
mushrooms, broccoli and mangetout;
simmer, uncovered, about 5 minutes
or until vegetables are tender.
4 Stir in onion, juice and sauce;
season to taste. Discard lime leaves
and chilli. Divide noodles into serving
bowls; ladle soup over noodles, top
with sprouts and herbs.

tip Reheat soup in a microwave on
HIGH (100%) for about 1½ minutes,
stirring halfway through heating.

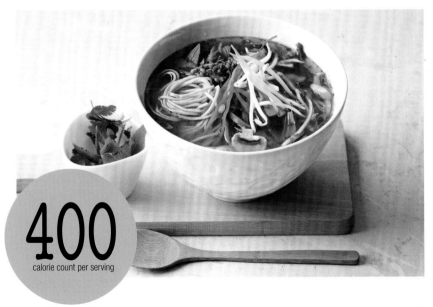

400
calorie count per serving

348 calorie count per serving

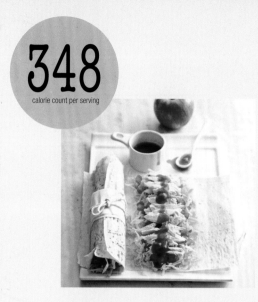

327 calorie count per serving

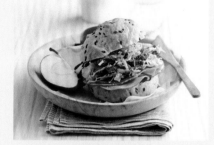

mexican chicken wrap

serves 2
prep time 10 minutes
nutritional count per serving 6.2g total fat
(2.1g saturated fat); 1455kJ (348 cal); 29.5g
carbohydrate; 40.8g protein; 4.7g fibre

2 thin wholemeal wraps
50g (2oz) finely shredded iceberg lettuce
40g (1½oz) reduced-fat cheddar cheese,
    coarsely grated
1 medium tomato (150g), finely chopped
100g (3½oz) skinless cooked chicken,
    shredded
60g (2oz) mild taco sauce
2 large apples (400g)

1 Place wraps on cutting board.
Spread lettuce along centre of each
wrap; top equally with cheese,
tomato, chicken and taco sauce.
Season. Roll to enclose filling.
2 Serve each wrap with an apple.

ham & basil coleslaw rolls

serves 2
prep time 10 minutes
nutritional count per serving 7.4g total
fat (1.7g saturated fat); 1367kJ (327 cal);
47g carbohydrate; 19.3g protein; 7.2g fibre

2 tablespoons extra-light mayonnaise
2 tablespoons fat-free natural yogurt
70g (2½oz) finely shredded cabbage
½ medium carrot (60g), coarsely grated
1 shallot (25g), thinly sliced
2 tablespoons torn fresh basil leaves
2 multigrain bread rolls
125g (4oz) wafer thin reduced-fat ham
2 large apples (400g)

1 Whisk mayonnaise and yogurt in
a medium bowl until combined. Mix
in cabbage, carrot, shallot and basil
leaves. Season.
2 Split rolls in half; sandwich
coleslaw and ham between rolls.
Serve each roll with an apple.

314

calorie count per serving

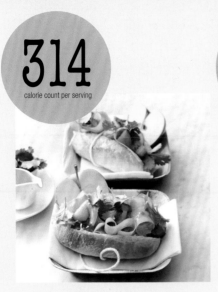

349

calorie count per serving

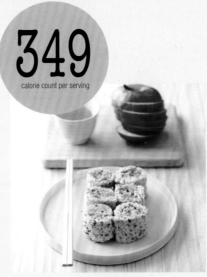

vietnamese-style vegetable roll

serves 2
prep time 10 minutes
nutritional count per serving 6g total fat
(1g saturated fat); 1313kJ (314 cal); 53.8g
carbohydrate; 7.2g protein; 7.7g fibre

½ cucumber (130g)
½ medium carrot (60g)
2 crusty long white bread rolls
2 tablespoons extra-light mayonnaise
50g (2oz) finely shredded iceberg lettuce
2 tablespoons sweet chilli sauce
4 tablespoons fresh coriander leaves
2 large apples (400g)

1 Slice cucumber and carrot into
ribbons. Split rolls lengthways,
without cutting all the way through.
2 Spread the base of each roll with
mayonnaise; top equally with lettuce,
carrot and cucumber. Drizzle sweet
chilli sauce between rolls and top with
coriander leaves. Season.
3 Serve each roll with an apple.

tuna sushi sandwiches

serves 2
prep time 10 minutes
nutritional count per serving 7.2g total fat
(2.8g saturated fat); 1459kJ (349 cal); 46.8g
carbohydrate; 19.8g protein; 9g fibre

95g (3½oz) canned tuna in springwater
½ medium carrot (60g)
½ cucumber (130g)
4 slices wholegrain bread
1½ tablespoons sweet chilli cream cheese
2 large apples (400g)

1 Drain and flake tuna. Cut carrot
and cucumber into matchsticks.
3 Remove crusts from bread. Using
a rolling pin, flatten bread. Spread
cream cheese over bread; place
tuna, cucumber and carrot in rows on
bread, leaving a 1cm (½-inch) border
along one edge. Season.
4 Roll bread from opposite edge to
enclose filling. Cut each roll into 3
rounds. Serve 6 rounds with an apple.

caesar salad with baked asparagus

serves 2
prep + cook time 35 minutes
nutritional count per serving 8.4g total fat
(1.9g saturated fat); 1488kJ (356 cal); 39.5g
carbohydrate; 23.6g protein; 11.8g fibre

3 slices rye bread (135g)
340g (12oz) asparagus, trimmed, halved
   diagonally
cooking oil spray
1 small courgette (90g)
95g (3½oz) fat-free natural yogurt
1 tablespoon lemon juice
2 teaspoons dijon mustard
1 well-drained anchovy fillet, chopped
   finely
2 romaine lettuce hearts
2 soft-boiled eggs, halved

1 Preheat oven to 180°C.
2 To make croûtons, remove crusts from bread; tear bread into small pieces. Place on baking-parchment-lined oven tray with asparagus; spray lightly with cooking oil. Bake about 10 minutes or until croûtons are crisp and asparagus is tender.
3 Meanwhile, using a vegetable peeler, slice courgette lengthways into thin ribbons. Combine yogurt, juice, mustard and anchovy in medium bowl.
4 Add courgette, lettuce and asparagus to yogurt mixture; mix gently. Season to taste. Serve salad topped with croûtons and egg.

tip If taking to work, pack the veggies and yogurt in separate containers; mix the veggies into the yogurt mixture at lunch time.

356
calorie count per serving

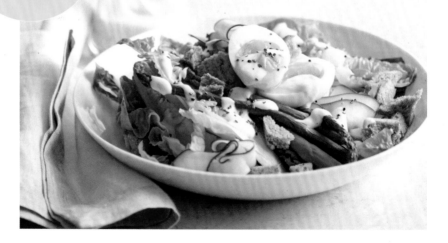

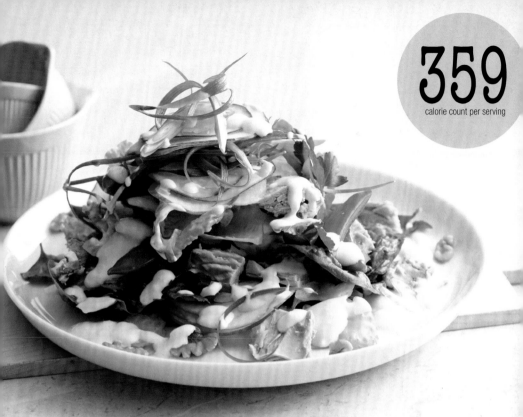

tuna waldorf salad

serves 2
prep + cook time 20 minutes
nutritional count per serving 7.3g total fat
(1.4g saturated fat); 1501kJ (359 cal); 27.7g
carbohydrate; 39.6g protein; 11g fibre

250g (8oz) sugar snap peas, trimmed
95g (3½oz) fat-free natural yogurt
1 tablespoon lemon juice
2 teaspoons dijon mustard
1 tablespoon water
1 large red apple (200g), unpeeled, cored,
　sliced thinly
2 stalks celery (300g), trimmed, sliced
　thinly
2 romaine lettuce hearts, leaves separated
　and torn
2 spring onions, sliced thinly
2 tablespoons finely chopped fresh flat-leaf
　parsley
3 x 95g (3½oz) cans tuna in springwater,
　drained, flaked
1 tablespoon walnuts, chopped coarsely

1 Boil, steam or microwave peas
until tender; drain. Rinse under cold
water; drain.
2 Combine yogurt, juice, mustard
and the water in medium bowl. Add
peas, apple, celery, lettuce, onion,
parsley and tuna; toss gently to
combine. Season to taste.
3 Divide salad between serving
plates; sprinkle with nuts.

tip If taking to work, pack the tuna
salad and the yogurt mixture in
separate containers; mix the yogurt
mixture into the salad at lunch time.

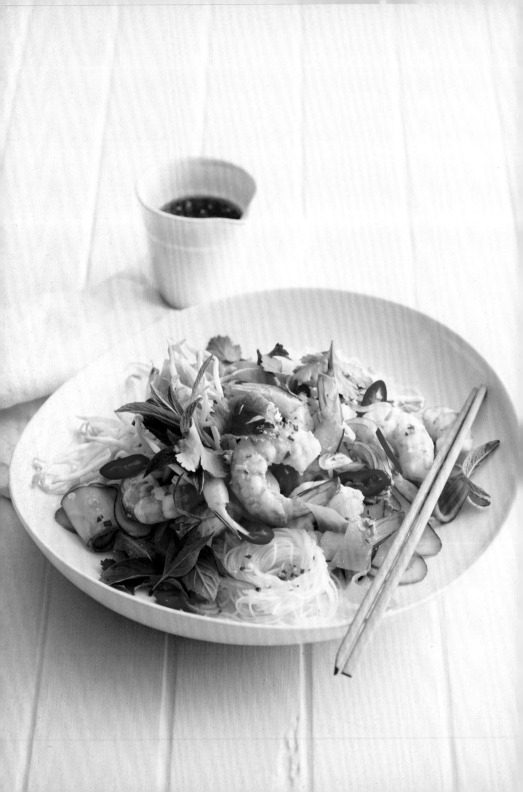

prawn & rice vermicelli salad

serves 2
prep time 35 minutes
nutritional count per serving 6.5g total fat
(0.9g saturated fat); 1476kJ (353 cal); 24g
carbohydrate; 45.9g protein; 5.4g fibre

100g (3½oz) rice vermicelli noodles
800g (1½lb) cooked medium prawns
1 large carrot (180g), cut into ribbons
½ cucumber (130g), cut into ribbons
1 fresh long red chilli, sliced thinly
80g (3oz) bean sprouts
2 purple shallots (50g), sliced thinly
3 tablespoons each fresh mint, coriander
   and thai basil leaves

chilli dressing
1 tablespoon light brown sugar
1 tablespoon fish sauce
2 tablespoons lime juice
1 fresh small red chilli, chopped finely
1 clove garlic, crushed
2 teaspoons olive oil

1 Place noodles in large heatproof
bowl, cover with boiling water; stand
until tender, drain. Return to bowl.
2 Meanwhile, shell and devein
prawns, leaving tails intact.
3 To make chilli dressing, combine
ingredients in screw-top jar; shake
well.
4 Add dressing, prawns and
remaining ingredients to noodles; mix
gently. Season to taste.

tip If taking this salad to work, pack
the dressing separately and add to
the salad at lunch time.

353

calorie count per serving

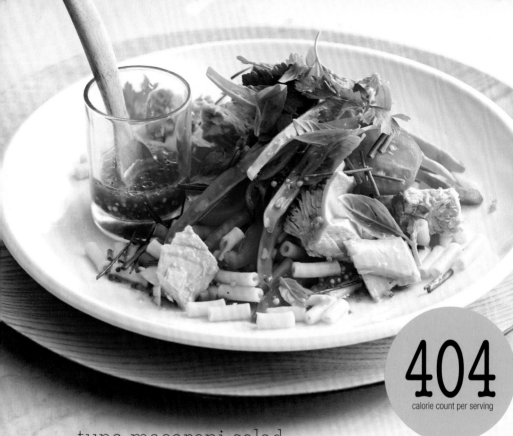

404
calorie count per serving

tuna macaroni salad

serves 2
prep + cook time 20 minutes
nutritional count per serving 7.6g total fat
(1.5g saturated fat); 1689kJ (404 cal); 51.3g
carbohydrate; 28.3g protein; 5.7g fibre

135g (5oz) macaroni
90g (3oz) green beans, trimmed, halved
  lengthways
1 fresh long red chilli, chopped finely
2 teaspoons olive oil
2 tablespoons red wine vinegar
2 teaspoons wholegrain mustard
1 tablespoon finely chopped fresh chives
1 tablespoon each fresh flat-leaf parsley
  and baby basil leaves
125g (4oz) cherry tomatoes, halved
1 small red pepper (150g), sliced thinly
180g (6oz) canned tuna in springwater,
  drained, flaked

1 Cook pasta in large saucepan of
boiling water until tender. Add beans
to pan for last 2 minutes of pasta
cooking time; drain. Rinse under cold
water; drain.
2 To make dressing, combine chilli,
oil, vinegar and mustard in small
bowl.
3 Combine pasta, beans, herbs,
tomato, pepper, tuna and dressing
in large bowl; toss gently. Season
to taste.

tip If taking to work, pack the salad
and dressing in separate containers;
mix the dressing into the salad at
lunch time.

spicy vegetable & lentil salad

serves 2
prep + cook time 50 minutes
nutritional count per serving 6.8g total fat
(0.9g saturated fat); 1622kJ (388 cal);
53.1g carbohydrate; 19.6g protein; 15g fibre

200g (7oz) baby carrots, trimmed
350g (12oz) pumpkin or butternut squash,
    cut into 2cm (¾-inch) wedges
1 medium red pepper (200g), sliced thickly
1 small red onion (100g), cut into wedges
1 medium courgette (120g), chopped
    coarsely
1 clove garlic, crushed
2 tablespoons balsamic vinegar
½ teaspoon dried chilli flakes
1 teaspoon cumin seeds, crushed lightly
400g (13oz) canned brown lentils, rinsed,
    drained
3 tablespoons finely chopped fresh
    coriander
50g (2oz) rocket leaves
2 teaspoons olive oil
1 small pitta bread (65g), halved
140g (5oz) fat-free natural yogurt

1 Preheat oven to 220°C. Line large baking dish with baking parchment.
2 Place carrots, pumpkin, pepper, onion, courgette, garlic, vinegar, chilli and cumin in dish; mix gently, season. Roast, uncovered, about 35 minutes or until vegetables are tender. Cool 10 minutes.
3 Combine vegetables in large bowl with lentils, coriander, rocket and oil; season to taste. Serve vegetable salad with bread and yogurt.

tip Make the salad close to serving so that the vegetables are still warm.

388
calorie count per serving

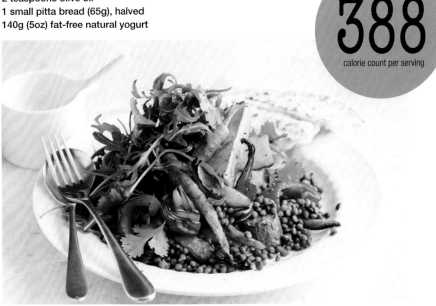

niçoise salad

serves 2
prep + cook time 35 minutes
nutritional count per serving 5.9g total fat
(1.7g saturated fat); 1484kJ (355 cal); 39.5g
carbohydrate; 30.3g protein; 9.1g fibre

8 baby new potatoes (320g), halved
175g (6oz) green beans, trimmed
60ml (2fl oz) fat-free french dressing
2 teaspoons dijon mustard
125g (4oz) baby plum tomatoes, halved
80g (3oz) pitted black olives
1 romaine lettuce heart, leaves separated
   and torn
1 hard-boiled egg, halved
180g (6oz) canned tuna in springwater,
   drained, flaked
2 well-drained anchovy fillets, halved
   lengthways

1 Boil, steam or microwave potato
and beans, separately, until tender;
drain. Rinse under cold water; drain.
2 Combine dressing and mustard
in large bowl. Add tomato, olives,
lettuce, egg, potato, beans and tuna;
mix gently. Season to taste. Serve
salad topped with anchovies.

tip If taking this salad to work, pack
the combined dressing and mustard
separately; toss the dressing through
the salad at lunch time.

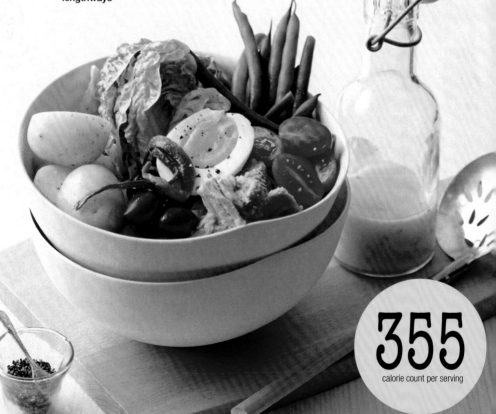

355
calorie count per serving

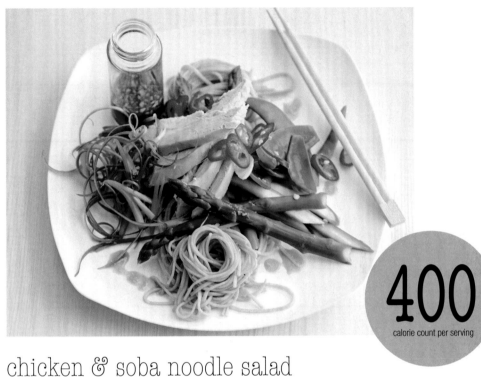

400
calorie count per serving

chicken & soba noodle salad

serves 2
prep + cook time 25 minutes
nutritional count per serving 5.1g total fat
(1.1g saturated fat); 1672kJ (400 cal); 46g
carbohydrate; 37.4g protein; 4.5g fibre

125g (4oz) dried soba noodles
170g (5½oz) asparagus, trimmed
60g (2oz) mangetout, trimmed
1 teaspoon sesame oil
1 tablespoon mirin
1 tablespoon rice wine vinegar
2 teaspoons japanese soy sauce
1 clove garlic, crushed
240g (8oz) cooked skinless chicken breast,
    thickly sliced
1 fresh long red chilli, sliced thinly
2 spring onions, shredded finely

1 Cook noodles in large saucepan of
boiling water until tender; drain.
2 Meanwhile, boil, steam or
microwave asparagus and
mangetout, separately, until tender;
drain. Rinse under cold water; drain.
3 To make dressing, combine oil,
mirin, vinegar, sauce and garlic
in small bowl. Combine chicken,
asparagus, mangetout, chilli, half
the onion, noodles and dressing in
large bowl; season to taste. Serve
sprinkled with remaining onion.

tip If taking to work, pack the
dressing separately; toss through the
salad at lunch time.

warm indian-style chicken salad

serves 2
prep + cook time 30 minutes
nutritional count per serving 8g total fat
(1.3g saturated fat); 1467kJ (351 cal); 33.8g
carbohydrate; 31.1g protein; 9.3g fibre

8 mini microwave pappadums (28g)
1 chicken breast fillet (200g)
1 teaspoon garam masala
2 medium carrots (240g), cut into ribbons
1 teaspoon sesame seeds, toasted
good handful each fresh coriander and
    mint leaves
2 purple shallots (50g), sliced thinly
60g (2oz) baby spinach leaves
1 fresh long red chilli, sliced thinly
40g (1½oz) sultanas

cumin dressing
½ teaspoon ground cumin
2 tablespoons lemon juice
2 teaspoons olive oil

351
calorie count per serving

1 Cook pappadums following
directions on the packet.
2 Slice chicken horizontally into four
thin slices; sprinkle garam masala
over both sides of chicken slices,
season. Cook chicken on heated
oiled griddle pan (or grill) until cooked
through.
3 Meanwhile, make cumin dressing:
Dry-fry cumin in small frying pan,
stirring, until fragrant. Combine cumin
and remaining ingredients in screw-
top jar; shake well.
4 Combine carrot, seeds, herbs,
shallot, spinach, chilli, sultanas and
dressing in medium bowl. Serve
chicken with salad; drizzle with
any remaining dressing. Serve with
pappadums.

tips Use a vegetable peeler to
slice the carrots lengthways into
thin ribbons. If taking to work,
pack chicken, salad and dressing
separately. At lunch time, reheat the
chicken, covered, in a microwave
oven on HIGH (100%) for about
1½ minutes. Toss the dressing
through the salad.

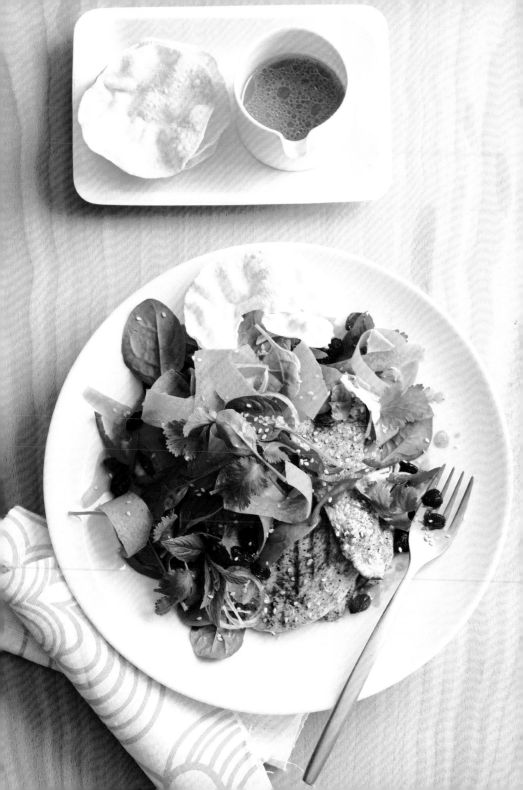

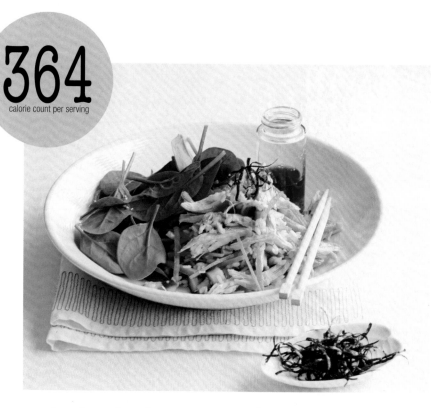

364 calorie count per serving

teriyaki chicken rice salad

serves 2
prep + cook time 35 minutes (+ standing)
nutritional count per serving 7.6g total fat
(1.8g saturated fat); 1522kJ (364 cal); 44.3g
carbohydrate; 26.2g protein; 3.7g fibre

100g (3½oz) sushi rice
180ml (6½fl oz) water
2 tablespoons rice vinegar
2 tablespoons teriyaki sauce
2cm (¾-inch) piece fresh ginger (10g),
    grated
160g (5½oz) skinless cooked chicken,
    shredded
½ cucumber (130g), chopped finely
1 medium carrot (120g), cut into
    matchsticks
60g (2oz) baby spinach leaves
2 teaspoons sesame seeds, toasted
½ sheet toasted seaweed (nori), shredded
    finely

1 Rinse rice with cold water until
water runs clear; drain well.
2 Combine rice and the water in
small saucepan, cover; bring to the
boil. Reduce heat; simmer, covered,
about 10 minutes or until rice is
tender. Remove from heat; stand rice,
covered, until cold.
3 Combine rice with vinegar, sauce
and ginger in large bowl. Add
chicken, cucumber, carrot, spinach
and seeds; toss gently to combine.
Season to taste. Serve rice salad
sprinkled with seaweed.

panzanella

serves 2
prep + cook time 20 minutes
nutritional count per serving 6.8g total fat
(0.9g saturated fat); 1480kJ (354 cal); 52g
carbohydrate; 15.5g protein; 10.8g fibre

1 small red pepper (150g)
1 small yellow pepper (150g)
2 medium tomatoes (300g), chopped
   coarsely
3 slices (110g) ciabatta bread, toasted, torn
½ small red onion (50g), sliced thinly
2 teaspoons rinsed, drained baby capers
50g (2oz) pitted black olives, halved
250g (8oz) canned mixed beans, rinsed,
   drained
3 tablespoons fresh small basil leaves
2 teaspoons olive oil
1 tablespoon red wine vinegar
1 clove garlic, crushed

1 Quarter peppers, discard
membranes and seeds. Place pepper,
skin-side up, on oven tray. Roast
under hot grill until skin blisters and
blackens. Cover pepper pieces in
plastic or paper for 5 minutes; peel
away skin, then slice thickly.
2 Meanwhile, place tomato in large
bowl; add bread, toss to combine.
3 Add pepper, onion, capers, olives,
beans, basil, oil, vinegar and garlic
to tomato mixture; toss gently to
combine. Season to taste.

tip Make the salad close to serving,
otherwise the bread will go soggy.
If taking to work, pack the bread
separately and toss through at lunch
time.

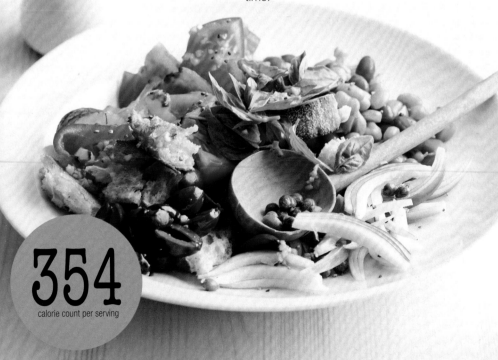

354
calorie count per serving

shredded vegetable rice paper rolls

serves 2
prep + cook time 25 minutes
nutritional count per serving 7.3g total fat
(1g saturated fat); 1463kJ (350 cal); 46g
carbohydrate; 18.4g protein; 12.8g fibre

½ medium red onion (85g), sliced thinly
1 large yellow pepper (350g), sliced thinly
150g (5oz) mangetout, trimmed, sliced
    thinly
120g (4oz) finely shredded chinese leaf
1 large carrot (180g), grated coarsely
50g (2oz) rice vermicelli noodles
½ cucumber (130g), cut into matchsticks
4 tablespoons each fresh mint and
    coriander leaves
6 x 22cm (9-inch) rice paper rounds
200g (7oz) piece marinated tofu, cut into
    6 slices, halved lengthways
125ml (4fl oz) sweet chilli sauce

350
calorie count per serving

1 Combine onion, pepper,
mangetout, cabbage and carrot
in medium bowl; cook mixture in
heated large non-stick frying pan,
over medium heat, stirring, about
5 minutes or until vegetables soften.
Strain mixture into colander over large
bowl; cool.

2 Meanwhile, place noodles in small
heatproof bowl, cover with boiling
water; stand until tender, drain. Chop
noodles coarsely.

3 Combine vegetable mixture
and noodles in medium bowl with
cucumber and herbs; season to
taste.

4 Dip one rice paper round into bowl
of warm water until soft. Lift sheet
from water; place on clean tea towel.
Top with one heaped tablespoon
of vegetable mixture and one slice
of tofu; drizzle with a little of the
sauce. Fold sheet over filling, then
fold in both sides. Continue rolling to
enclose filling.

5 Repeat step 4 to make a total of
six rolls.

6 Serve rolls with remaining sauce.

tip Keep the rolls moist by covering
them with a slightly damp piece of
absorbent paper, then store them in
an airtight container in the refrigerator.

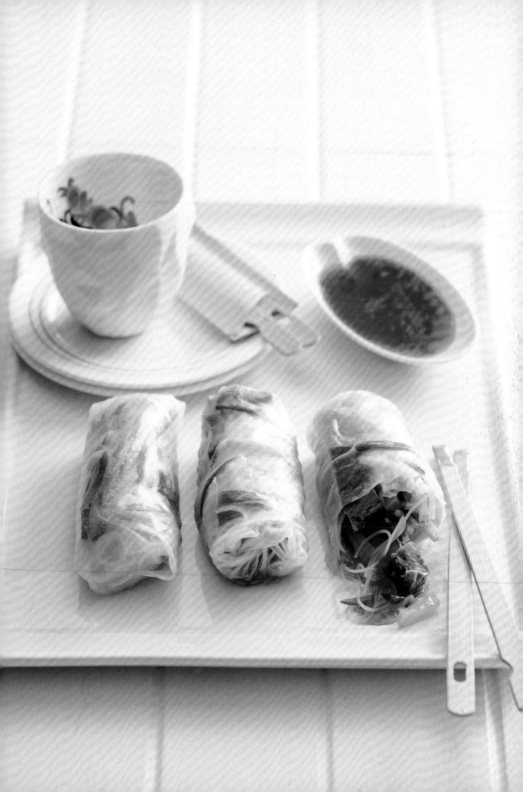

sweet potato hummus with vegetables

serves 2
prep + cook time 45 minutes
nutritional count per serving 7.3g total fat
(3.2g saturated fat); 1509kJ (361 cal); 53g
carbohydrate; 16.9g protein; 7.5g fibre

1 small sweet potato (250g), chopped
   coarsely
cooking oil spray
½ teaspoon ground cumin
1 large pitta bread (80g)
125g (4oz) canned chickpeas, rinsed,
   drained
1 clove garlic, crushed
2 tablespoons lemon juice
60ml (2fl oz) water
80g (3oz) pitted mixed olives
125g (4oz) cherry tomatoes, cut in half
½ cucumber (130g), cut into wedges
60g (2oz) reduced-fat feta cheese, cut into
   2cm (¾-inch) slices

1 Preheat oven to 200°C. Line oven
tray with baking parchment.
2 Place sweet potato on tray; spray
lightly with cooking oil, sprinkle with
cumin, season. Roast sweet potato
about 25 minutes or until tender; add
pitta bread to tray for last 5 minutes
of sweet potato cooking time. Cool
5 minutes.
3 Blend or process sweet potato,
chickpeas, garlic, juice and the water
until almost smooth. Season to taste.
Serve sweet potato hummus with
bread and remaining ingredients.

361
calorie count per serving

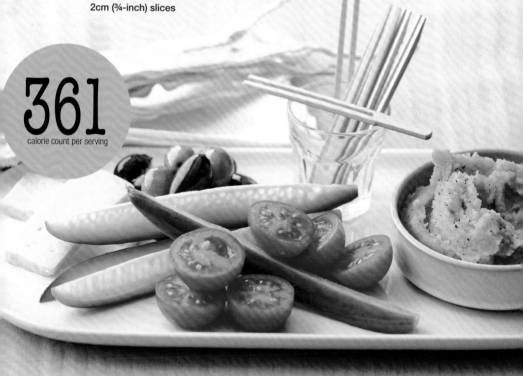

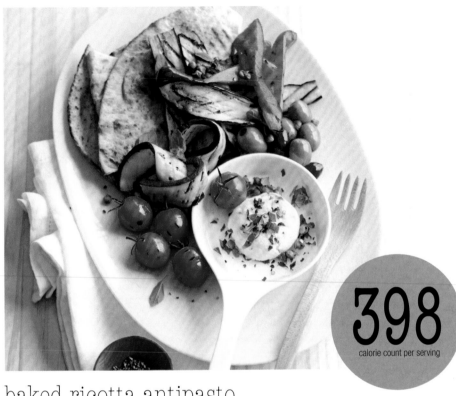

398
calorie count per serving

baked ricotta antipasto

serves 2
prep + cook time 30 minutes
nutritional count per serving 9g total fat
(4.1g saturated fat); 1664kJ (398 cal); 57.1g
carbohydrate; 16.2g protein; 11.5g fibre

100g (3½oz) ricotta
cooking oil spray
pinch dried chilli flakes
2 teaspoons coarsely chopped fresh
   oregano
1 medium courgette (120g), sliced thinly
4 baby aubergines (240g), sliced thinly
1 medium red pepper (200g), sliced thickly
125g (4oz) cherry tomatoes
2 large pitta bread (160g)
80g (3oz) pitted mixed olives
1 tablespoon rinsed, drained capers

1 Preheat oven to 180°C. Line oven
tray with baking parchment.
2 Shape cheese into 2 rounds,
place on tray; spray with cooking
oil, sprinkle with chilli and half the
oregano. Bake cheese about
20 minutes or until heated through.
3 Meanwhile, cook courgette,
aubergine, pepper, tomatoes and
bread, in batches, on heated oiled
griddle pan (or grill) until vegetables
are tender and bread is crisp.
4 Sprinkle ricotta with remaining
oregano; serve immediately with
vegetables, bread, olives and capers.

primavera frittata

serves 2
prep + cook time 35 minutes
nutritional count per serving 7.9g total fat
(2.8g saturated fat); 1496kJ (358 cal); 34.5g
carbohydrate; 31.7g protein; 10g fibre

1 large brown onion (200g), chopped finely
2 cloves garlic, crushed
2 medium potatoes (400g), trimmed,
  chopped coarsely
170g (6oz) asparagus, chopped coarsely
2 medium courgettes (240g), sliced thinly
2 eggs
6 egg whites
80ml (3fl oz) skimmed milk
4 tablespoons finely chopped fresh herbs
  (see tips)
60g (2oz) frozen peas
1½ tablespoons finely grated parmesan
  cheese
1 tablespoon fresh dill sprigs

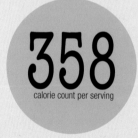

358
calorie count per serving

1 Heat medium (20cm/8 inch base) non-stick frying pan over medium heat; cook onion and garlic, stirring, about 10 minutes or until onion is browned lightly.

2 Meanwhile, boil, steam or microwave potato, asparagus and courgettes, separately, until tender; drain.

3 Whisk eggs, egg whites, milk and herbs in medium jug; season.

4 Add potato, asparagus and courgettes to pan. Pour egg mixture over vegetables; sprinkle with peas. Reduce heat to low; cook, uncovered, about 10 minutes or until frittata is almost set. Sprinkle with cheese.

5 Preheat grill. Grill frittata about 2 minutes or until set. Stand frittata in pan 5 minutes before serving sprinkled with dill.

tips We used a mixture of parsley, basil and dill for this recipe, but you can use any herbs you like. If your frying pan does not have a heatproof handle, cover the handle with aluminium foil to protect it from the heat of the grill. Frittata can be served warm or cold. Reheat slices of frittata, covered, in a microwave on HIGH (100%) for about 1½ minutes.

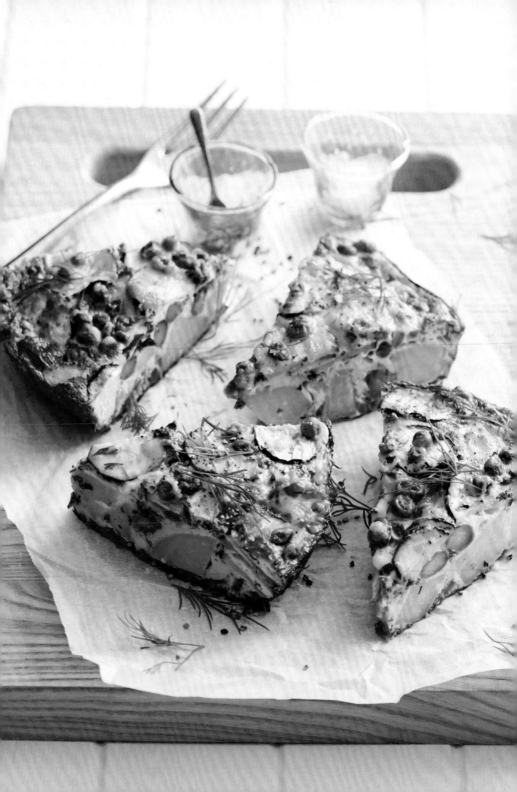

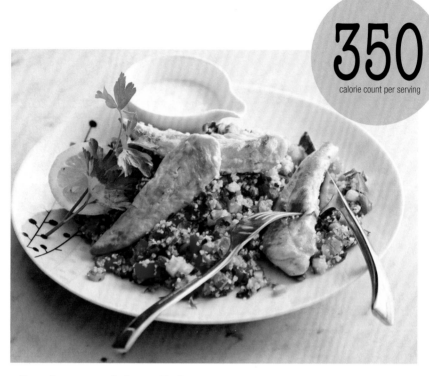

350 calorie count per serving

chicken tabbouleh

serves 2
prep + cook time 20 minutes
nutritional count per serving 7.4g total fat
(1.7g saturated fat); 1463kJ (350 cal); 29.9g
carbohydrate; 58.8g protein; 9g fibre

80g (3oz) bulgur wheat
6 chicken mini fillets (450g)
2 medium tomatoes (300g), chopped finely
½ cucumber (130g), chopped finely
3 spring onions, sliced thinly
good handful finely chopped fresh flat-leaf
  parsley
2 tablespoons lemon juice
1 clove garlic, crushed
95g (3½oz) fat-free natural yogurt
1 lemon, cut into wedges

1 Dry-fry bulgur wheat in large
non-stick frying pan over medium
heat, stirring, about 2 minutes or until
browned lightly. Transfer to medium
heatproof bowl. Cover bulgur wheat
with boiling water; stand about
10 minutes or until it is tender. Drain
bulgur wheat; squeeze out excess
liquid, return to bowl.
2 Cook chicken in same heated pan
over medium heat.
3 To make tabbouleh; stir tomato,
cucumber, onion, parsley, juice and
garlic into bulgur wheat; season to
taste. Serve tabbouleh with chicken,
yogurt and lemon wedges.

tip The chicken can be reheated
in a microwave, covered, on HIGH
(100%), for about 1½ minutes.

ham, egg & vegetable fried rice

serves 2
prep + cook time 20 minutes
nutritional count per serving 7.8g total fat
(2.2g saturated fat); 1505kJ (360 cal);
47.1g carbohydrate; 21.2g protein; 8.1g fibre

1 teaspoon rice bran oil
1 egg, beaten lightly
1 small brown onion (100g), chopped finely
90g (3oz) green beans, chopped coarsely
1 clove garlic, crushed
90g (3½oz) wafer-thin reduced-fat ham,
   sliced thinly
75g (3oz) small oyster mushrooms
1 small carrot (70g), sliced thinly
60g (2oz) frozen peas
250g (8oz) cold cooked brown long-grain
   rice
1 tablespoon kecap manis
1 spring onion, shredded finely

1 Heat half the oil in wok; pour egg into wok, tilt wok to make a thin omelette; cook until set. Remove omelette from wok; roll tightly, then slice thinly.

2 Heat remaining oil in wok; stir-fry brown onion, beans and garlic until onion just softens. Add ham, mushrooms, carrot and peas; stir-fry about 3 minutes or until mushrooms are tender.

3 Add rice and kecap manis; stir-fry until hot. Season to taste. Toss omelette and spring onion through rice just before serving.

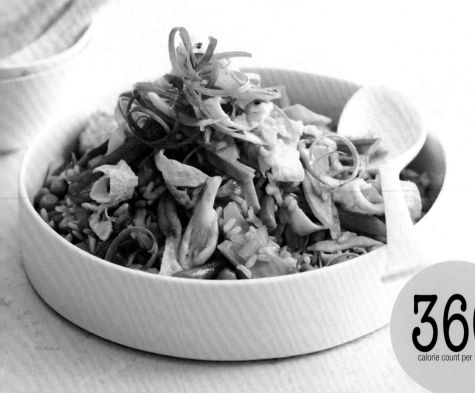

360
calorie count per serving

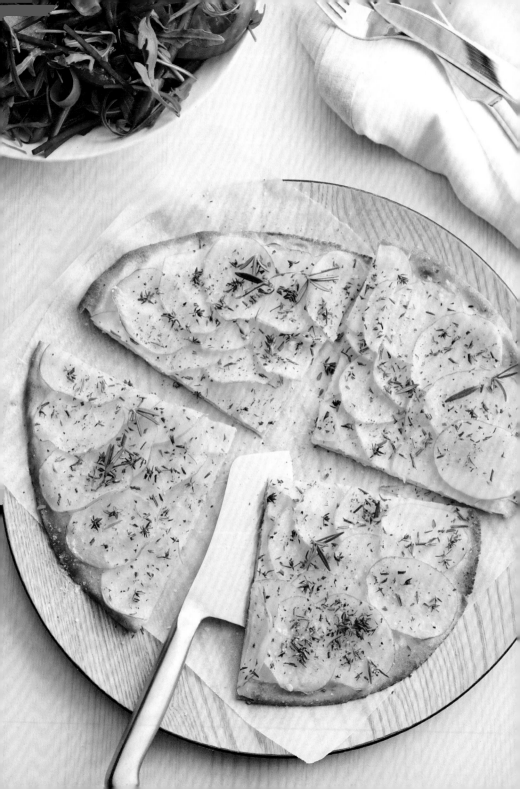

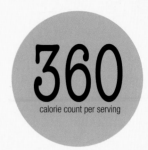

360
calorie count per serving

potato & rosemary pizza with garden salad

serves 2
prep + cook time 25 minutes
nutritional count per serving 7.9g total fat
(1.9g saturated fat); 1505kJ (360 cal); 50.9g
carbohydrate; 14.2g protein; 12.2g fibre

2 medium potatoes (400g), sliced thinly
1 large pitta bread (80g)
2 teaspoons garlic-infused olive oil
1½ tablespoons finely grated parmesan
    cheese
3 teaspoons finely chopped fresh rosemary
2 teaspoons fresh thyme leaves

garden salad
125g (4oz) green beans, trimmed
125g (4oz) rocket, trimmed
1 medium tomato (150g), sliced thinly
1 medium carrot (120g), cut into ribbons
1 small fresh beetroot (100g), peeled, cut
    into matchsticks
1 tablespoons balsamic vinegar

1 Boil, steam or microwave potato
until tender; drain.
2 Preheat oven to 220°C. Line oven
tray with baking parchment.
3 Place bread on tray; brush with
half the oil. Sprinkle with cheese;
arrange potato slices, slightly
overlapping, over cheese. Sprinkle
pizza with herbs; drizzle with
remaining oil, season. Bake pizza
about 15 minutes or until base is
crisp.
4 Meanwhile, make garden salad:
Boil, steam or microwave beans
until tender; drain. Rinse under cold
water; drain. Combine beans, rocket,
tomato, carrot, beetroot and vinegar
in large bowl; season to taste.
5 Serve pizza with salad.

tip Use disposable gloves when
handling beetroot to stop it from
staining your hands. This recipe is
best served immediately.

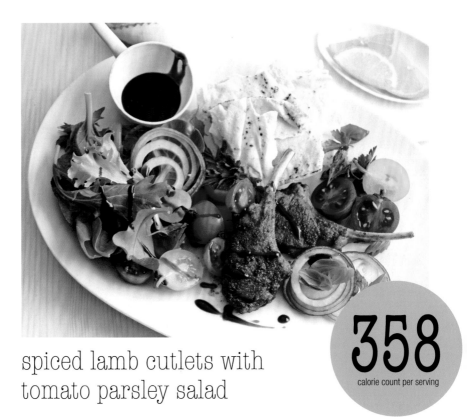

spiced lamb cutlets with tomato parsley salad

358 calorie count per serving

serves 2
prep + cook time 20 minutes
nutritional count per serving 7.1g total fat
(2.2g saturated fat); 1496kJ (358 cal); 49.4g
carbohydrate; 19.3g protein; 6.9g fibre

1 teaspoon ground cumin
2 teaspoons each ground coriander and
   paprika
4 french-trimmed lamb cutlets (200g)
400g (13oz) mixed baby tomatoes, halved
½ small red onion (50g), sliced thinly
2 tablespoons each fresh flat-leaf parsley
   and small basil leaves
1 tablespoon lemon juice
60g (2oz) mixed salad leaves
1 tablespoon balsamic glaze
2 large pitta bread (160g), toasted, torn into
   pieces
1 lemon, cut into wedges

1 Combine spices in a small bowl;
sprinkle spice mixture over both sides
of cutlets.
2 Heat large non-stick frying pan
over medium heat; cook cutlets until
cooked as desired.
3 Meanwhile, combine tomato,
onion, herbs and juice in small bowl;
season to taste. Place salad leaves
in another small bowl; drizzle over
balsamic glaze.
4 Serve lamb with salads, bread and
lemon.

tip The cutlets can be reheated,
covered, in a microwave oven on
HIGH (100%), for about 1½ minutes.

courgette burger

serves 2
prep + cook time 40 minutes
nutritional count per serving 5.1g total fat
(1.2g saturated fat); 1651kJ (395 cal);
65.2g carbohydrate; 17.1g protein; 8.5g fibre

2 medium courgettes (240g), grated
   coarsely
35g (1½oz) packaged breadcrumbs
1 tablespoon finely grated parmesan
   cheese
1 spring onion, sliced thinly
1 egg white, beaten lightly
1 tablespoon finely chopped fresh flat-leaf
   parsley
cooking oil spray
1 large brown onion (200g), sliced thinly
4 small lettuce leaves
1 small fresh beetroot (100g), peeled,
   grated coarsely
2 tablespoons tomato relish
2 hamburger buns (180g), split, toasted

1 Place courgette in strainer;
squeeze out excess water. Combine
courgette, breadcrumbs, cheese,
onion, egg white and parsley in
medium bowl; season. Shape mixture
into two patties.

2 Spray medium frying pan with
cooking oil; cook onion, stirring,
about 10 minutes or until browned
lightly. Remove from pan.

3 Cook patties in same pan until
browned both sides and heated
through.

4 Sandwich lettuce, patties, onion,
beetroot and relish between bun
halves.

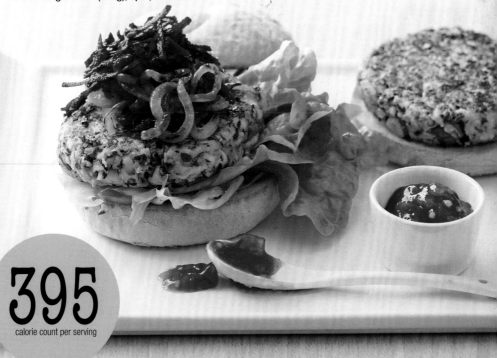

395
calorie count per serving

chilli jam lamb with char-grilled vegetables

serves 2
prep + cook time 45 minutes
nutritional count per serving 7.5g total fat
(2.1g saturated fat); 1601kJ (383 cal); 30.4g
carbohydrate; 41.7g protein; 10.4g fibre

1 tablespoon chilli jam
60ml (2fl oz) lemon juice
200g (7oz) lamb fillet
1 medium red pepper (200g), sliced thickly
170g (5½oz) asparagus, trimmed, halved
2 medium courgettes (240g), sliced thickly
4 baby aubergines (240g), sliced thickly
60g (2oz) baby spinach leaves
1 small pitta bread (65g), cut into wedges

mint sauce
1 clove garlic, crushed
1 tablespoon finely chopped fresh mint
80ml (3fl oz) fat-free natural yogurt

1 To make mint sauce, combine
ingredients in small bowl.
2 Combine chilli jam and
1 tablespoon of the lemon juice in
medium bowl; add lamb, turn to coat,
season. Cook lamb on heated oiled
griddle pan (or grill) until cooked as
desired. Cover lamb; stand 5 minutes
then slice thinly.
3 Meanwhile, combine pepper,
asparagus, courgette, aubergine
and remaining lemon juice in large
bowl; cook vegetables, in batches,
on griddle pan until tender. Return
vegetables to bowl with spinach; toss
gently to combine. Season to taste.
4 Serve lamb with vegetables and
bread; drizzle with mint sauce.

tip This recipe is best served
immediately.

383

calorie count per serving

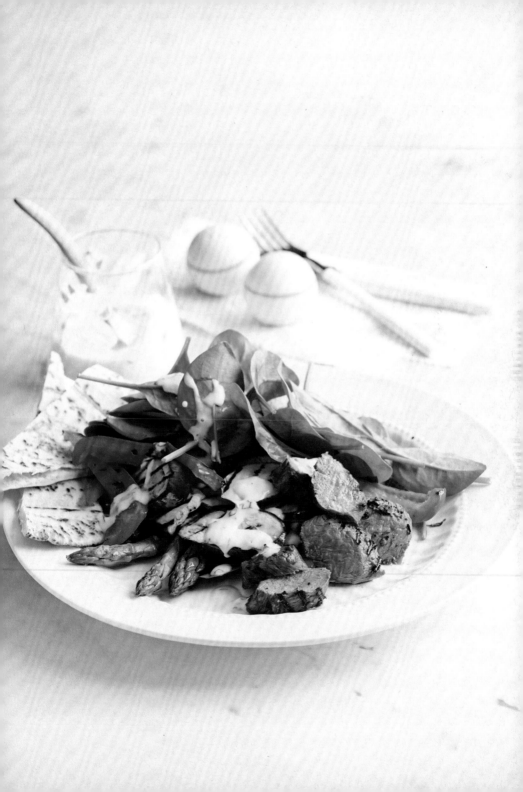

salmon bruschetta

serves 2
prep time 20 minutes
nutritional count per serving 8.1g total fat
(2.9g saturated fat); 1501kJ (359 cal); 42.1g
carbohydrate; 26.1g protein; 5.4g fibre

4 slices ciabatta bread (140g)
1 clove garlic, halved
100g (3½oz) rocket leaves
2 spring onions, sliced thinly
1 small fresh beetroot (100g), peeled, cut
    into matchsticks
2 teaspoons balsamic glaze
40g (1½oz) reduced-fat onion and chive
    cream cheese
½ cucumber (130g), cut into ribbons
4 slices smoked salmon (120g)
2 teaspoons fresh dill sprigs

1 Toast bread; rub one side of toasts
with garlic.
2 Meanwhile, to make rocket salad,
combine half the rocket with onion,
beetroot and balsamic glaze in
medium bowl. Season to taste.
3 Spread toasts with cream cheese
and top with remaining rocket,
cucumber and salmon; sprinkle with
dill and serve with rocket salad.

tips Use a vegetable peeler to slice
the cucumber lengthways into thin
ribbons. Use disposable gloves when
handling beetroot to prevent staining
your fingers.

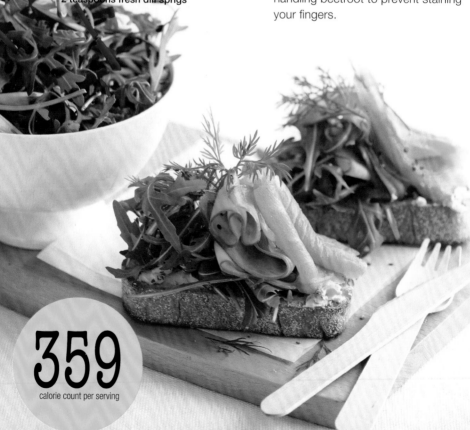

359
calorie count per serving

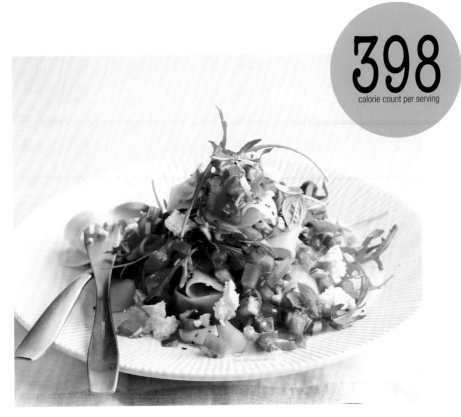

398
calorie count per serving

pappardelle with fresh tomato sauce

serves 2
prep + cook time 25 minutes
nutritional count per serving 4.9g total fat
(2.2g saturated fat); 1664kJ (398 cal); 64.2g
carbohydrate; 17.5g protein; 9.1g fibre

1 medium red onion (170g), chopped finely
2 cloves garlic, crushed
3 tablespoons coarsely chopped fresh
   basil
1 tablespoon red wine vinegar
5 medium tomatoes (750g), chopped finely
150g (5oz) pappardelle pasta
60g (2oz) rocket leaves
60g (2oz) ricotta, crumbled

1 Combine onion, garlic, basil,
vinegar and tomato in medium bowl;
stand 10 minutes.
2 Meanwhile, cook pasta in large
saucepan of boiling water until
tender; drain. Return pasta to pan;
add tomato mixture and rocket, mix
gently. Season to taste.
3 Serve pasta topped with cheese.

tips This recipe is best served
immediately.

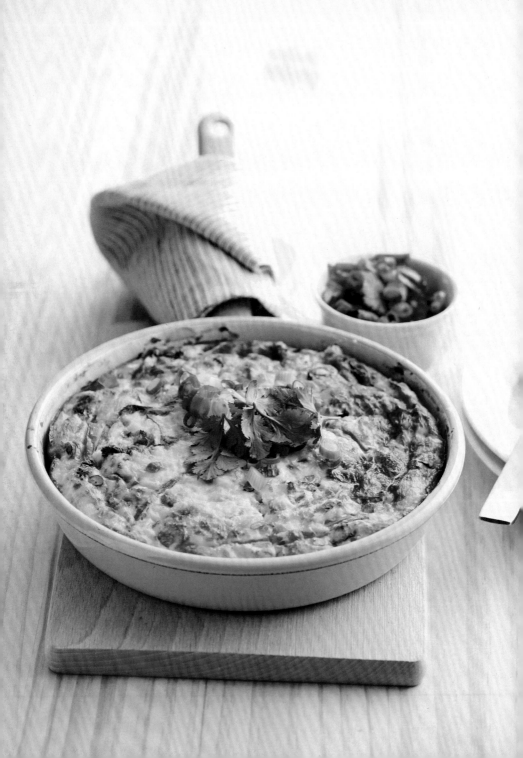

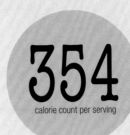

354 calorie count per serving

mexican-style tortilla

serves 2
prep + cook time 1 hour
nutritional count per serving 7g total fat
(2.3g saturated fat); 1480kJ (354 cal);
39.7g carbohydrate; 29.4g protein; 7g fibre

1 medium (400g) sweet potato, chopped
   coarsely
2 eggs
6 egg whites
80ml (3fl oz) skimmed milk
125g (4oz) canned creamed corn
80g (3oz) roasted red pepper, coarsely
   chopped
2 large tomatoes (440g), deseeded, sliced
   thinly
3 spring onions, sliced thinly
3 tablespoons fresh coriander leaves
25g (1oz) reduced-fat cheddar cheese,
   coarsely grated

1 Preheat oven to 180°C. Line oven tray with baking parchment.
2 Place sweet potato on tray; roast about 30 minutes or until tender.
3 Meanwhile, whisk eggs, egg whites, milk and corn in medium jug until combined; season.
4 Heat medium non-stick frying pan (20cm/8 inch base) over medium heat; place sweet potato, pepper, tomato, half the onion and half the coriander in pan. Pour egg mixture over vegetables, reduce heat to low; cook, uncovered, about 10 minutes or until tortilla is almost set.
5 Preheat grill. Sprinkle tortilla with cheese; grill about 2 minutes or until cheese melts and tortilla is set. Stand tortilla in pan 5 minutes before sprinkling with remaining onion and coriander to serve.

tips If your frying pan does not have a heatproof handle, cover the handle with aluminium foil to protect it from the heat of the grill. The tortilla can be served warm or cold. Reheat tortilla slices, covered, in a microwave on HIGH (100%) for about 1½ minutes.

mains

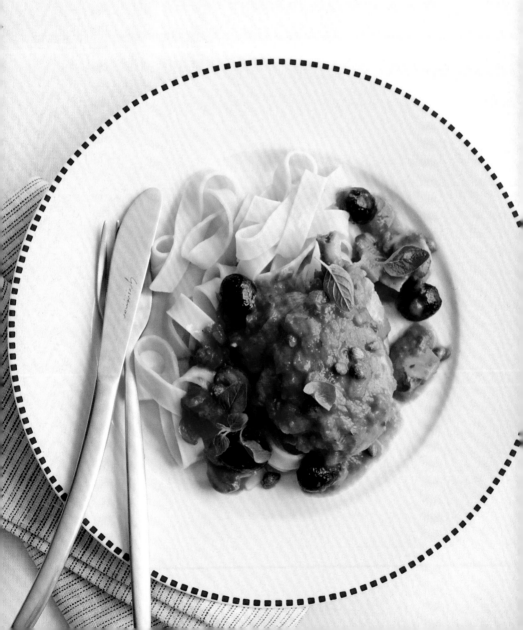

chicken cacciatore

serves 2 **prep + cook time** 50 minutes
nutritional count per serving 8g total fat (2g saturated fat);
1672kJ (400 cal); 59.3g carbohydrate; 28.3g protein; 7.1g fibre

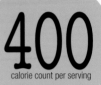

400
calorie count per serving

2 skinless chicken drumsticks (260g)
100g (3½oz) small button mushrooms, sliced thickly
1 small brown onion (100g), chopped finely
1 slice prosciutto (15g), chopped coarsely
1 clove garlic, crushed
2 anchovy fillets, well-drained, chopped finely
60ml (2fl oz) dry white wine
260g (9oz) bottled tomato pasta sauce
100g (3½oz) fettuccine pasta
60g (2oz) pitted black olives
1 tablespoon rinsed, drained baby capers
1½ tablespoons fresh oregano leaves

1 Heat large non-stick saucepan over medium heat; cook chicken,
turning, until browned all over.
2 Add mushrooms, onion, prosciutto, garlic and anchovies to pan; cook,
stirring occasionally, about 5 minutes or until onion softens. Add wine; bring
to the boil. Reduce heat, stir in sauce; simmer, covered, turning chicken
occasionally, about 25 minutes or until chicken is cooked through.
3 Meanwhile, cook pasta in large pan of boiling water until tender; drain.
4 Add olives, capers and half the oregano to chicken; simmer,
uncovered, about 5 minutes. Season to taste.
5 Serve chicken and sauce with pasta;
sprinkle with remaining oregano.

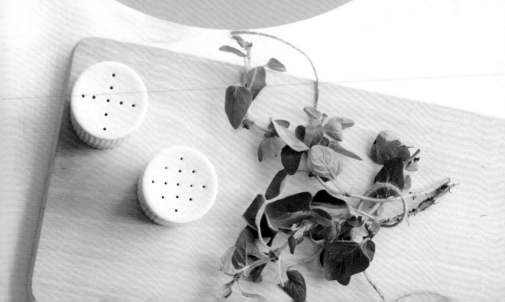

sweet chilli chicken stir-fry

serves 2
prep + cook time 25 minutes
nutritional count per serving 3.8g total fat
(1g saturated fat); 1672kJ (400 cal); 45.1g
carbohydrate; 41.9g protein; 6.8g fibre

65g (2½oz) jasmine rice
300g (10oz) chicken breast fillets, sliced
    thinly
1 small red onion (100g), cut into thin
    wedges
4cm (1½-inch) piece fresh ginger (20g),
    grated
1 large carrot (180g), sliced thinly
1 medium red pepper (200g), sliced thinly
60ml (2fl oz) water
150g (5oz) sugar snap peas, trimmed
60ml (2fl oz) sweet chilli sauce
2 tablespoons japanese soy sauce
3 tablespoons fresh coriander leaves

1 Bring medium saucepan of water
to the boil, gradually add rice; boil,
uncovered, about 20 minutes or until
rice is tender, drain.
2 Meanwhile, combine chicken,
onion and ginger in medium bowl.
Heat lightly oiled wok; stir-fry chicken
mixture, in batches, until chicken is
browned and onion softens. Remove
from wok.
3 Add carrot, pepper and the water
to wok; stir-fry until carrot is almost
tender. Return chicken mixture to wok
with peas and sauces; stir-fry until
vegetables are tender. Season
to taste.
4 Serve stir-fry with rice; sprinkle
with coriander.

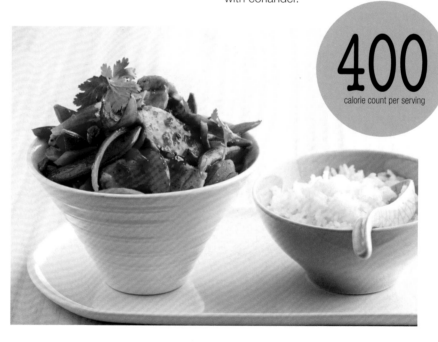

400
calorie count per serving

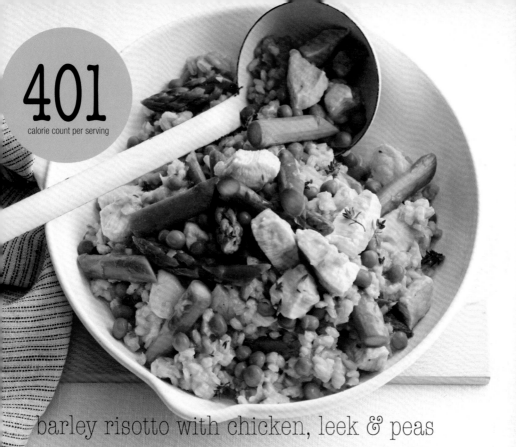

barley risotto with chicken, leek & peas

serves 2
prep + cook time 55 minutes
nutritional count per serving 6.2g total fat
(1.3g saturated fat); 1676kJ (401 cal); 43.2g
carbohydrate; 36.4g protein; 14.1g fibre

560ml (17½fl oz) chicken stock
1 teaspoon olive oil
1 large leek (500g), sliced thinly
2 cloves garlic, crushed
2 sprigs fresh thyme
100g (3½oz) pearl barley
200g (7oz) chicken breast fillet, chopped
    coarsely
170g (5½oz) asparagus, chopped coarsely
60g (2oz) frozen peas

1 Bring stock to the boil in medium
pan. Reduce heat; simmer, covered.
2 Heat oil in medium pan; cook
leek, garlic and thyme, stirring, until
leek softens. Add barley; stir to coat
in leek mixture. Stir in 250ml (8fl oz)
simmering stock; cook, stirring, over
low heat until liquid is absorbed.
Continue adding simmering stock in
125ml (4fl oz) batches, stirring, until
liquid is absorbed after each addition.
Total cooking time should be about
35 minutes or until barley is tender.
3 Stir in chicken, asparagus and peas;
cook, covered, stirring occasionally,
about 5 minutes or until chicken is
cooked and asparagus is tender.
Discard thyme. Season to taste.

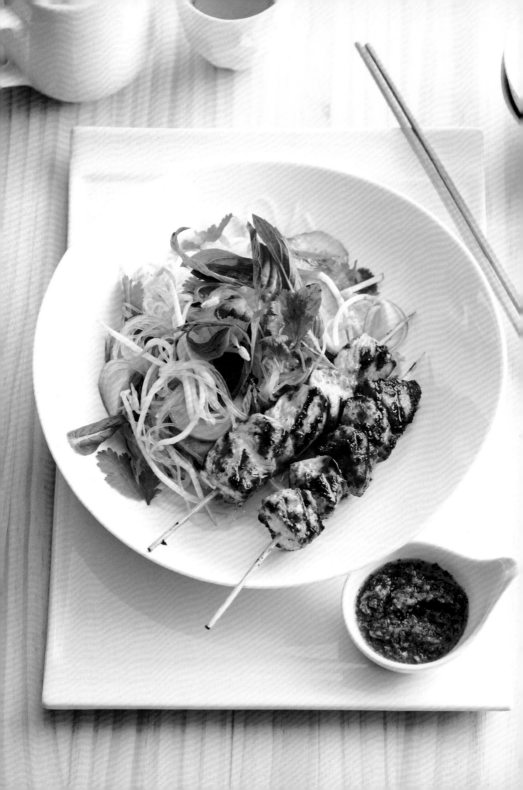

nam jim chicken with rice noodle salad

serves 2
prep + cook time 45 minutes
nutritional count per serving 8.3g total fat
(1.7g saturated fat); 1643kJ (393 cal); 28.5g
carbohydrate; 49g protein; 3.4g fibre

2 tablespoons grated palm sugar
1 teaspoon each ground cumin and
    coriander
2 chicken breast fillets (400g), chopped
    coarsely

nam jim
1 clove garlic, chopped coarsely
2 fresh long green chillies, chopped
    coarsely
1 fresh coriander root
6 tablespoons fresh coriander leaves
1 tablespoon fish sauce
1 tablespoon grated palm sugar
1 purple shallot (25g), chopped coarsely
1½ tablespoons lime juice

noodle salad
50g (2oz) rice vermicelli noodles
½ cucumber (130g), cut into matchsticks
80g (3oz) bean sprouts
2 purple shallots (50g), sliced thinly
4 tablespoons each fresh mint, coriander
    and thai basil leaves
2 teaspoons fish sauce
1 tablespoon lime juice
1 teaspoon olive oil

1 To make nam jim, blend or process
ingredients until smooth. Transfer half
the nam jim to shallow dish; stir in the
sugar and spices.
2 Thread chicken onto four skewers;
coat chicken in nam jim mixture.
Cook skewers on heated oiled griddle
pan (or grill) until chicken is cooked.
3 Meanwhile, make noodle salad:
place noodles in large heatproof
bowl, cover with boiling water; stand
until tender, drain. Return to bowl.
Add remaining ingredients; toss
gently. Season to taste.
4 Serve skewers with salad and
remaining nam jim.

tips Soak wooden skewers in water
for at least 30 minutes before using
to prevent them from burning during
cooking. If you have time, refrigerate
the marinated skewers, covered, for
30 minutes before cooking.

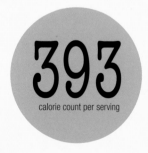

393
calorie count per serving

moroccan fish kebabs with couscous salad

serves 2
prep + cook time 45 minutes
nutritional count per serving 1.5g total fat
(0.3g saturated fat); 1605kJ (384 cal); 48.5g
carbohydrate; 40.4g protein; 3.2g fibre

300g (10oz) firm white fish fillets, chopped
   coarsely
1½ tablespoons moroccan seasoning
100g (3½oz) couscous
125ml (4fl oz) boiling water
1 medium orange (240g), segmented
3 tablespoons coarsely chopped fresh
   flat-leaf parsley
30g (1oz) baby spinach leaves

coriander yogurt
95g (3½oz) fat-free natural yogurt
1 tablespoon lemon juice
1 teaspoon garam masala
¼ teaspoon chilli powder
1 clove garlic, crushed
2 tablespoons finely chopped fresh
   coriander

1 To make coriander yogurt, combine ingredients in small bowl.
2 Thread fish onto four skewers; sprinkle seasoning all over skewers. Cook skewers on heated oiled griddle pan (or grill) until fish is cooked.
3 Meanwhile, combine couscous with the water in large heatproof bowl, cover; stand about 5 minutes or until liquid is absorbed, fluffing with fork occasionally. Stir in orange, parsley and spinach; season to taste.
4 Serve skewers with couscous salad and yogurt.

tips Soak wooden skewers in water for at least 30 minutes before using to prevent them from burning during cooking. You can use any firm white fish fillets for this recipe.

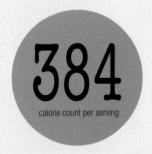

384
calorie count per serving

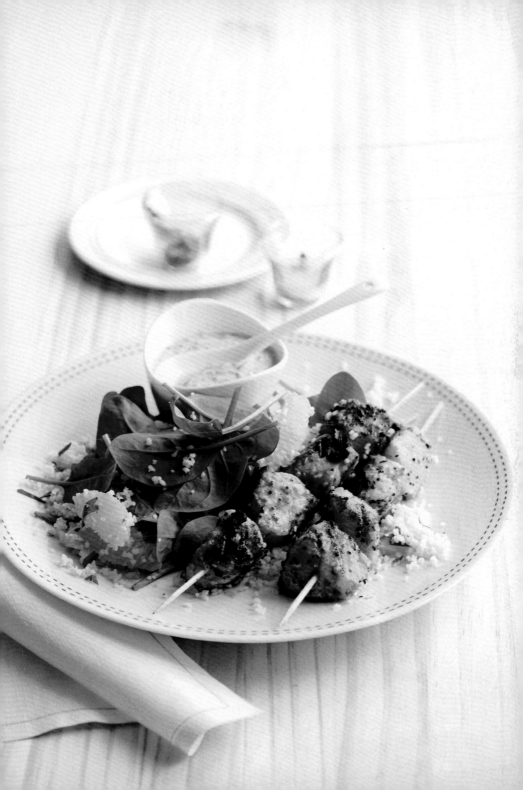

szechuan-style prawns with rice noodles

serves 2
prep + cook time 40 minutes (+ refrigeration)
nutritional count per serving 3.9g total fat
(0.4g saturated fat); 1680kJ (402 cal); 48.8g
carbohydrate; 36.6g protein; 10.5g fibre

500g (1lb) uncooked medium prawns
2 teaspoons szechuan peppercorns
¼ teaspoon paprika
1 clove garlic, crushed
2 tablespoons light soy sauce
2 tablespoons hoisin sauce
60ml (2fl oz) vegetable or fish stock
1 tablespoon lemon juice
80ml (3fl oz) water
1 fresh small red chilli, chopped finely
200g (7oz) thick fresh rice noodles
1 small white onion (100g), sliced thinly
1 medium red pepper (200g), sliced thickly
115g (3½oz) fresh baby corn, halved
    lengthways
500g (1lb) bok choy, chopped coarsely
2 spring onions, shredded finely

1 Shell and devein prawns, leaving
tails intact.
2 Using mortar and pestle, crush
peppercorns until fine; transfer to
medium bowl. Add paprika, garlic,
sauces, stock, juice, 1 tablespoon
of the water and chilli. Add prawns
to peppercorn mixture; mix gently.
Cover; refrigerate 3 hours.
3 Place noodles in small heatproof
bowl, cover with boiling water; stand
until tender, drain.
4 Remove prawns from marinade,
reserve marinade. Heat lightly oiled
wok; stir-fry prawns, in batches, until
changed in colour. Remove from wok.
5 Add white onion, pepper, corn and
the remaining water to wok; stir-fry
about 5 minutes or until vegetables
are tender. Return prawns to wok with
reserved marinade, noodles, bok choy
and spring onion; stir-fry until sauce
comes to the boil. Season to taste.

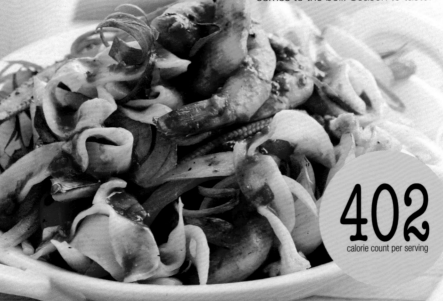

402
calorie count per serving

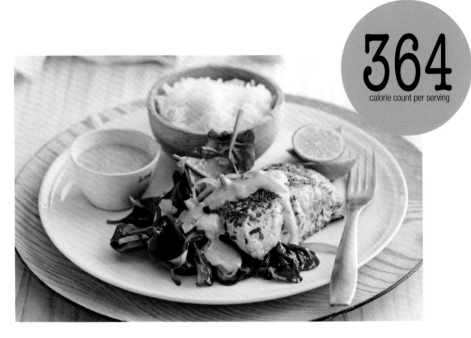

kerala-style fish with lime pickle yogurt

serves 2
prep + cook time 50 minutes (+ refrigeration)
nutritional count per serving 8.1g total fat
(2.1g saturated fat); 1522kJ (364 cal);
24.8g carbohydrate; 45.6g protein; 1.7g fibre

1 teaspoon each coriander and cumin
 seeds
2 cardamom pods, bruised
1 cinnamon stick
½ teaspoon ground turmeric
¼ teaspoon chilli powder
2 teaspoons groundnut oil
1 clove garlic, crushed
2 x 200g (7oz) firm white fish fillets
50g (2oz) basmati rice
½ small red onion (50g), sliced thinly
80g (3oz) baby spinach leaves
70g (2½oz) fat-free natural yogurt
1 tablespoon lime pickle, chopped finely
1 tablespoon lime juice
1 lime, cut into wedges

1 Dry-fry spices in small frying pan,
stirring, until fragrant. Using mortar
and pestle, crush until fine; transfer
to medium bowl. Add oil, garlic and
fish; turn to coat fish in spice mixture.
Cover; refrigerate 30 minutes.
2 Bring medium saucepan of water
to the boil, gradually add rice; boil,
uncovered, about 20 minutes or until
rice is tender, drain.
3 Meanwhile, cook fish in medium
non-stick frying pan over medium heat
until cooked as desired. Remove from
pan; cover to keep warm.
4 Cook onion in same pan, stirring,
until softened. Add spinach; cook,
stirring, until spinach is wilted. Season
to taste.
5 Combine yogurt, pickle and juice
in small bowl. Serve fish with spinach
mixture, yogurt and lime wedges.

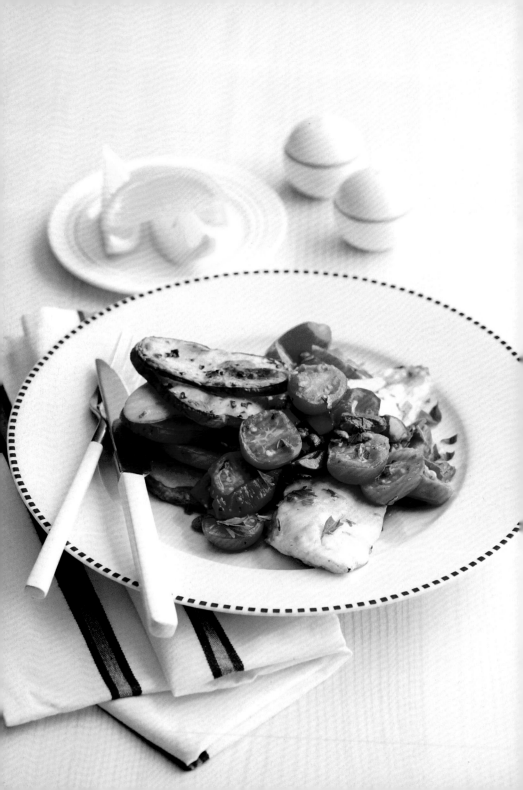

baked fish fillets with chilli potatoes

serves 2
prep + cook time 1 hour
nutritional count per serving 3.2g total fat
(1g saturated fat); 1576kJ (377 cal); 42g
carbohydrate; 39.6g protein; 7.2g fibre

3 medium potatoes (600g), cut into 1cm
   (½-inch) slices
125ml (4fl oz) chicken stock
¼ teaspoon dried chilli flakes, crushed
½ teaspoon sea salt flakes
2 x 150g (5oz) firm white fish fillets
½ medium lemon (70g), cut into wedges

tomato & caper salsa
250g (8oz) cherry tomatoes, halved
120g (4oz) drained roasted red pepper,
   chopped coarsely
1 tablespoon lemon juice
2 tablespoons pitted black olives, chopped
   finely
1 tablespoon rinsed, drained baby capers
2 tablespoons finely chopped fresh flat-leaf
   parsley

377
calorie count per serving

1 Preheat oven to 180°C.
2 Place potato, in a single layer, in
lightly oiled baking dish. Pour stock
over potatoes; bake, uncovered
30 minutes or until liquid is almost
absorbed.
3 Meanwhile, make tomato and
caper salsa: place tomato on
baking-paper-lined oven tray; bake,
alongside potato, about 15 minutes
or until softened. Cool 5 minutes.
Combine tomato, pepper, juice,
olives, capers and parsley in medium
bowl; season.
4 Increase oven to 240°C. Remove
potato from oven; sprinkle with
chilli and salt. Place fish on baking-
parchment-lined oven tray; season.
Bake fish and potato about
15 minutes or until potato is browned
lightly and fish is cooked.
5 Serve fish with salsa, potato and
lemon wedges.

tips We used snapper for this
recipe, but use any firm white fish
fillets you like.

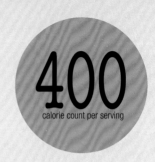

thai-style fish cakes with cucumber chilli pickle

serves 2
prep + cook time 40 minutes
nutritional count per serving 2.3g total fat
(0.2g saturated fat); 1672kJ (400 cal); 64.9g
carbohydrate; 33.4g protein; 4.3g fibre

125g (4oz) rice vermicelli noodles
250g (8oz) firm white fish fillets, chopped
    coarsely
6 tablespoons fresh coriander leaves
2 tablespoons cornflour
1 tablespoon fish sauce
1 tablespoon sweet chilli sauce
1 egg white, beaten lightly
2 spring onions, sliced thinly
30g (1oz) green beans, trimmed, sliced
    thinly
60g (2oz) mixed salad leaves

cucumber chilli pickle
2 tablespoons white wine vinegar
2 teaspoons caster sugar
1 clove garlic, crushed
1 fresh small red chilli, chopped finely
¼ teaspoon sea salt flakes
½ cucumber (130g), halved lengthways,
    sliced thinly
1 purple shallot (25g), sliced thinly
2 tablespoons fresh coriander leaves

1 Place noodles in small heatproof bowl, cover with boiling water; stand until tender, drain. Chop noodles coarsely.

2 To make cucumber chilli pickle, combine vinegar, sugar, garlic, chilli and salt in medium bowl; stir until sugar dissolves. Add cucumber, shallot and coriander; toss gently together. Combine pickle with half the noodles in medium bowl; season to taste.

3 Process fish until almost smooth. Add coriander, cornflour, sauces and egg white; process until combined. Stir in onion, beans and the remaining noodles; season. Shape mixture into six patties.

4 Heat medium non-stick frying pan over medium heat; cook patties about 3 minutes each side or until browned both sides and cooked through. Serve fish cakes with salad leaves and cucumber chilli pickle noodles.

tips You can use any firm white fish fillets for this recipe.

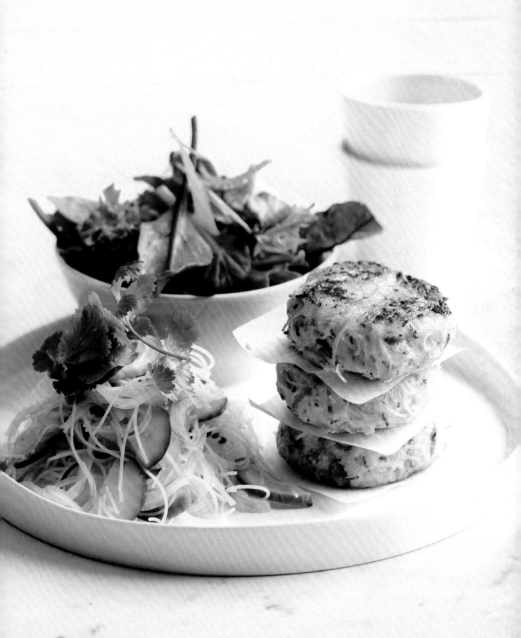

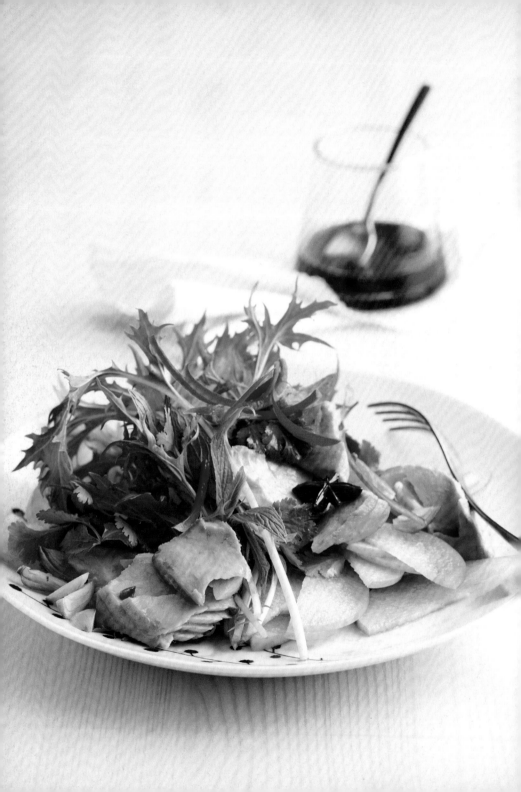

honey spiced salmon with nashi pear salad

serves 2
prep + cook time 35 minutes
nutritional count per serving 8.1g total fat
(1.7g saturated fat); 1530kJ (366 cal); 46.5g
carbohydrate; 23.1g protein; 4.4g fibre

1 teaspoon dried pink peppercorns,
  crushed
1 star anise
1 tablespoon japanese soy sauce
2 tablespoons honey
cooking oil spray
200g (7oz) skinless salmon fillet
2 medium nashi pears (400g), unpeeled,
  sliced thinly
1 fresh long red chilli, sliced thinly
2 purple shallots (50g), sliced thinly
4 tablespoons each fresh coriander and
  mint leaves
60g (2oz) mizuna

sesame dressing
¼ teaspoon sesame oil
1 tablespoon mirin
1 tablespoon rice wine vinegar
2 tablespoons japanese soy sauce

1 Preheat oven to 180°C.
2 Dry-fry spices in small frying pan, stirring, until fragrant. Add sauce and honey; bring to the boil. Reduce heat; simmer, uncovered, 1 minute.
3 Line small shallow baking dish with foil, extending foil 5cm (2 inches) above long sides of dish; spray with cooking oil. Place fish on foil; brush both sides of fish with honey mixture. Cover dish with foil; roast about 10 minutes or until fish is cooked as desired. When cool enough to handle, flake fish into large pieces.
4 Meanwhile, make sesame dressing: combine ingredients in screw-top jar; shake well. Season to taste.
5 Combine remaining ingredients with dressing in medium bowl. Serve fish with salad.

tips Nashi pears, also known as Asian pears, have a flavour that is a mix of apple and pear. If you can't find them, you can use the same weight of apples or pears. If you can't find mizuna, use rocket leaves instead.

366
calorie count per serving

chermoulla lamb with chickpea salad

serves 2
prep + cook time 45 minutes
nutritional count per serving 6.9g total fat
(2.1g saturated fat); 1672kJ (400 cal); 41.6g
carbohydrate; 36.7g protein; 8.5g fibre

200g (6½oz) lamb fillet
1 large pitta bread (80g)
250g (8oz) canned chickpeas, rinsed,
　　drained
½ small red onion (50g), sliced thinly
2 medium tomatoes (300g), cut into thin
　　wedges
2 tablespoons each fresh mint and
　　coriander leaves
60g (2oz) rocket leaves, shredded coarsely
2 tablespoons lemon juice
95g (3½oz) fat-free natural yogurt
½ medium lemon (70g), cut into wedges

chermoulla
handful coarsely chopped fresh coriander
6 tablespoons coarsely chopped fresh
　　flat-leaf parsley
1 clove garlic, crushed
1 teaspoon each ground cumin and
　　paprika
2 tablespoons lemon juice
2 tablespoons water

1 To make chermoulla, blend or
process ingredients until smooth.
2 Reserve half the chermoulla.
Combine remaining chermoulla and
lamb in medium bowl; season.
3 Cook lamb and bread on heated
oiled griddle pan (or grill) until lamb is
cooked as desired and bread is crisp.
Cover lamb; stand 5 minutes then
slice thinly. Break bread into pieces.
4 Meanwhile to make salad,
combine chickpeas, onion, tomato,
herbs, rocket and juice in medium
bowl; season to taste.
5 Divide salad between serving
plates; top with lamb and reserved
chermoulla. Serve with bread, yogurt
and lemon wedges.

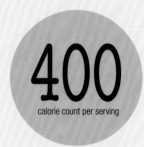

400
calorie count per serving

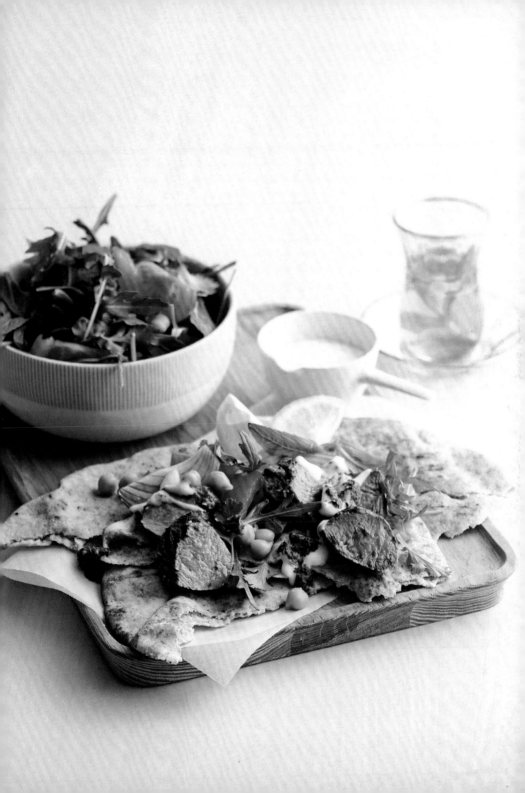

five-spice lamb and chilli stir-fry with greens

serves 2
prep + cook time 30 minutes
nutritional count per serving 8.3g total fat
(3.3g saturated fat); 1551kJ (371 cal); 12.4g
carbohydrate; 55.6g protein; 11.5g fibre

400g (13oz) lamb fillet, sliced thinly
1 teaspoon five-spice powder
2 cloves garlic, crushed
1 small red onion (100g), cut into thin
    wedges
80ml (3fl oz) water
175g (6oz) tenderstem broccoli, chopped
    coarsely
250g (8oz) sugar snap peas, trimmed
150g (5oz) oyster mushrooms, chopped
    coarsely
2 tablespoons hot chilli sauce
2 tablespoons japanese soy sauce
1 fresh long red chilli, sliced thinly

1 Combine lamb and five-spice in medium bowl.
2 Heat lightly oiled wok; stir-fry lamb, in batches, until browned. Remove from wok.
3 Add garlic and onion to wok; stir-fry about 5 minutes or until onion softens. Add 60ml (2fl oz) of the water, broccoli, peas and mushrooms; stir-fry until vegetables are tender.
4 Return lamb to wok with the remaining water and sauces; stir-fry until hot. Season to taste. Serve stir-fry sprinkled with chilli.

371 calorie count per serving

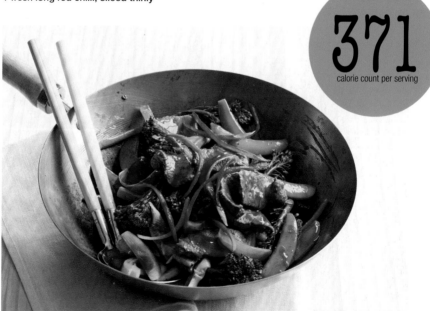

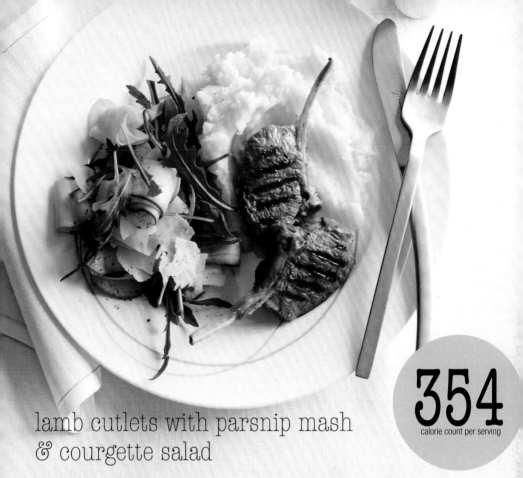

lamb cutlets with parsnip mash & courgette salad

354 calorie count per serving

serves 2
prep + cook time 45 minutes
nutritional count per serving 8g total fat
(2.6g saturated fat); 1480kJ (354 cal);
41.3g carbohydrate; 24g protein; 8.1g fibre

2 medium potatoes (400g), chopped
   coarsely
1 large parsnip (350g), chopped coarsely
125ml (4fl oz) skimmed milk, warmed
1 teaspoon olive oil
1 teaspoon finely grated lemon rind
1½ tablespoons lemon juice
1 tablespoon flaked parmesan cheese
1 large green courgette (150g), cut into
   ribbons
1 large yellow courgette (150g), cut into
   ribbons
40g (1½oz) rocket leaves
4 french-trimmed lamb cutlets (200g)

1 Boil, steam or microwave potato
and parsnip until tender; drain. Mash
potato and parsnip with milk in large
bowl until smooth; season to taste.
Cover to keep warm.
2 Meanwhile, combine oil, rind and
juice in medium bowl; add cheese,
courgette and rocket, mix gently.
Stand 15 minutes. Season to taste.
3 Cook lamb on heated oiled griddle
pan (or grill) until cooked as desired.
4 Serve lamb with mash and
courgette salad.

tip Use a vegetable peeler to slice the
courgette lengthways into thin ribbons.

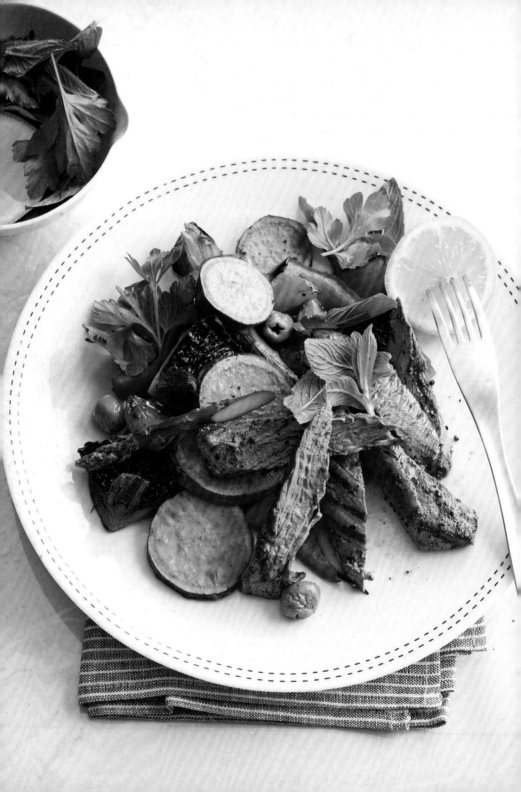

grilled pepper lamb with roast vegetables

serves 2
prep + cook time 55 minutes
nutritional count per serving 7.3g total fat
(2.5g saturated fat); 1651kJ (395 cal); 33.6g
carbohydrate; 43.6g protein; 8.7g fibre

1 small sweet potato (250g), unpeeled,
   sliced thinly
4 shallots (100g), quartered
1 large red pepper (350g), sliced thickly
2 flat mushrooms (160g), quartered
2 sprigs fresh rosemary
80g (3oz) pitted green olives
cooking oil spray
170g (5½oz) asparagus, halved
300g (10oz) lamb fillets
1 teaspoon coarse ground black pepper
2 tablespoons lemon juice
4 tablespoons each fresh flat-leaf parsley
   and mint leaves
1 medium lemon (140g), cut into wedges

1 Preheat oven to 200°C.

2 Combine sweet potato, shallot,
pepper, mushrooms, rosemary and
olives in large baking dish. Spray
with cooking oil; season, mix gently.
Roast, uncovered, about 35 minutes
or until vegetables are tender, adding
asparagus to dish for last 15 minutes
of cooking time. Discard rosemary.

3 Meanwhile, combine lamb and
pepper in small bowl. Cook lamb
on heated oiled griddle pan (or grill)
until cooked as desired. Cover lamb;
stand 5 minutes then slice thickly.

4 Stir juice and herbs into vegetable
mixture. Serve lamb with vegetables
and lemon wedges.

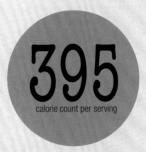

395
calorie count per serving

beef with black bean sauce

serves 2
prep + cook time 45 minutes
nutritional count per serving 7.6g total fat
(2.6g saturated fat); 1522kJ (364 cal); 43.1g
carbohydrate; 28.7g protein; 6.3g fibre

65g (2½oz) jasmine rice
1 teaspoon cornflour
2 tablespoons water
60ml (2fl oz) black bean sauce
200g (7oz) lean beef fillet, sliced thinly
2 cloves garlic, crushed
1 medium white onion (170g), cut into thin
   wedges
1 medium green pepper (200g), sliced
   thickly
1 large carrot (180g), halved, sliced into
   batons
2 stalks celery (300g), trimmed, sliced into
   batons
60ml (2fl oz) water, extra
2 spring onions, chopped coarsely

1 Bring medium saucepan of water
to the boil, gradually add rice; boil
uncovered about 20 minutes or until
rice is tender, drain.
2 Blend cornflour with the water and
sauce in small bowl.
3 Heat lightly oiled wok; stir-fry beef,
in batches, until browned. Remove
from wok.
4 Add garlic, white onion, pepper,
carrot, celery and the extra water to
wok; stir-fry about 5 minutes or until
vegetables are tender. Return beef
to wok with cornflour mixture; stir-fry
until sauce boils and thickens.
5 Remove from heat; stir in spring
onion. Season to taste. Serve stir-fry
with rice.

tip Add black bean sauce to taste
as different brands vary in thickness,
saltiness and taste.

364
calorie count per serving

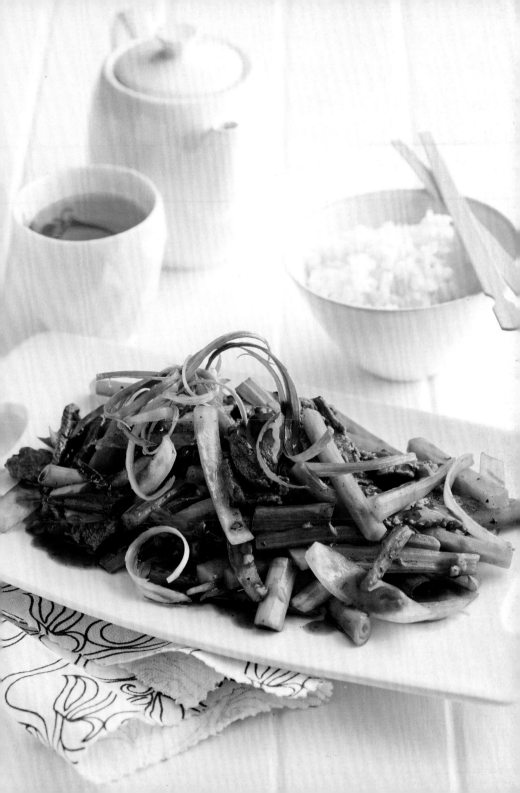

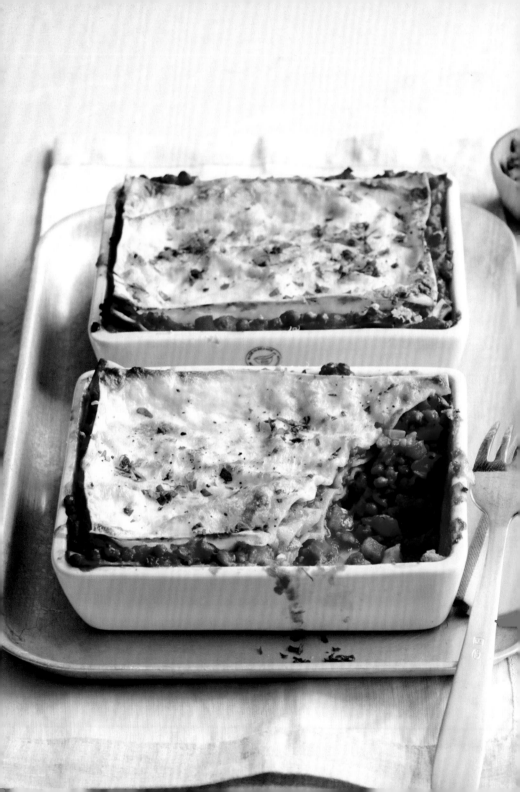

beef & lentil lasagne

serves 2
prep + cook time 1 hour 35 minutes
nutritional count per serving 6.6g total fat
(2.5g saturated fat); 1668kJ (399 cal); 52g
carbohydrate; 32.7g protein; 7.9g fibre

1 small red onion (100g), chopped finely
2 cloves garlic, crushed
1 small red pepper (150g), chopped finely
150g (5oz) lean minced beef
200g (7oz) canned brown lentils, rinsed,
   drained
1 teaspoon dried oregano
125ml (4fl oz) water
400g (13oz) canned chopped tomatoes
1 tablespoon cornflour
160ml (5½fl oz) skimmed milk
2 fresh lasagne sheets, cut into thirds
1½ tablespoons finely grated parmesan
   cheese
2 tablespoons finely chopped fresh
   flat-leaf parsley

1 Heat medium non-stick saucepan over medium heat; cook onion and garlic, stirring, about 5 minutes or until onion softens. Add pepper and beef; cook, stirring, about 5 minutes or until beef is browned. Add lentils, oregano, the water and undrained tomatoes; bring to the boil. Reduce heat; simmer, uncovered, about 15 minutes or until sauce thickens. Season to taste.

2 Preheat oven to 180°C. Lightly oil two shallow 500ml (17fl oz) ovenproof dishes.

3 Blend cornflour with 60ml (2fl oz) of the milk in small jug. Bring remaining milk to the boil in small saucepan; stir in cornflour mixture. Cook, stirring, until white sauce boils and thickens.

4 Spoon 4 tablespoons of meat sauce between dishes; top each with a pasta sheet, trimming to fit. Divide one-quarter of the remaining meat sauce between dishes; top each with a pasta sheet. Repeat layering with remaining meat sauce; top with remaining pasta sheet. Spread white sauce evenly over each dish; sprinkle each with cheese.

5 Bake lasagnes for about 50 minutes or until pasta is tender and cheese is browned lightly. Serve sprinkled with parsley.

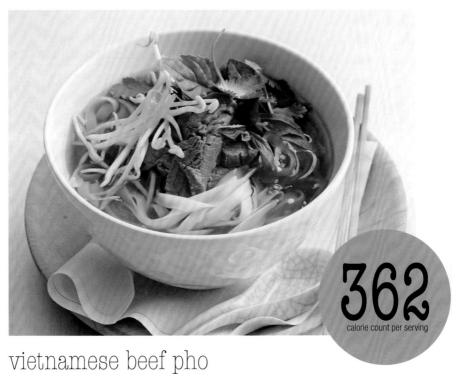

vietnamese beef pho

serves 2
prep + cook time 40 minutes
nutritional count per serving 7.5g total fat
(2.9g saturated fat); 1513kJ (362 cal); 34.9g
carbohydrate; 36.6g protein; 3g fibre

1 litre (1¾ pints) salt-reduced beef stock
6cm (2½-inch) piece fresh ginger (30g),
    sliced thinly
1 small brown onion (100g), sliced thinly
1 clove garlic, quartered
1 star anise
1 cinnamon stick
1 tablespoon grated palm sugar
1 tablespoon fish sauce
175g (6oz) dried rice stick noodles
200g (7oz) beef eye fillet, sliced thinly
40g (1½oz) bean sprouts
1 fresh long red chilli, sliced thinly
3 tablespoons each fresh mint, coriander
    and thai basil leaves

1 Combine stock, ginger, onion, garlic, star anise, cinnamon, sugar and sauce in large saucepan; bring to the boil. Reduce heat; simmer, covered, 20 minutes. Strain broth through fine sieve into large heatproof bowl; discard solids.

2 Return broth to pan; bring to the boil. Add noodles; simmer, uncovered, about 5 minutes or until noodles are tender. Add beef; return to the boil. Remove from heat.

3 Ladle soup into serving bowls; top with sprouts, chilli and herbs.

beef with red wine sauce & sweet potato crush

serves 2
prep + cook time 45 minutes
nutritional count per serving 7.8g total fat
(3.2g saturated fat); 1672kJ (400 cal); 33.7g
carbohydrate; 40.2g protein; 6.5g fibre

300g (10oz) piece lean beef fillet
3 teaspoons plain flour
125ml (4fl oz) beef stock
60ml (2fl oz) red wine
150g (5oz) trimmed watercress
1 tablespoon horseradish cream

sweet potato crush
1 medium sweet potato (450g), unpeeled
2 tablespoons orange juice
1 teaspoon fresh thyme leaves

1 Preheat oven to 200°C.
2 Make sweet potato crush: boil,
steam or microwave sweet potato
until tender; cool. Peel and coarsely
crush sweet potato with the back of
a fork, or a potato masher, in medium
saucepan. Add juice and thyme;
gently stir over medium heat until hot.
Season to taste.
3 Meanwhile, heat lightly oiled small
flameproof baking dish on stove top;
cook beef, turning, until browned
all over. Transfer to oven, roast,
uncovered, about 20 minutes or until
cooked to your liking. Remove from
dish, cover with foil; stand 10 minutes.
4 Place baking dish over medium
heat on stove top. Add flour; cook,
stirring, until mixture bubbles and
thickens. Gradually add stock and
wine; cook, stirring, until sauce boils
and thickens. Strain sauce into small
heatproof jug. Season to taste.
5 Serve sliced beef with watercress,
horseradish cream, sauce and sweet
potato crush.

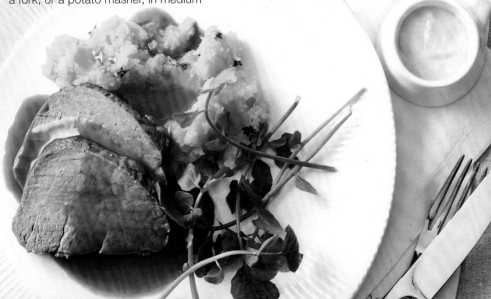

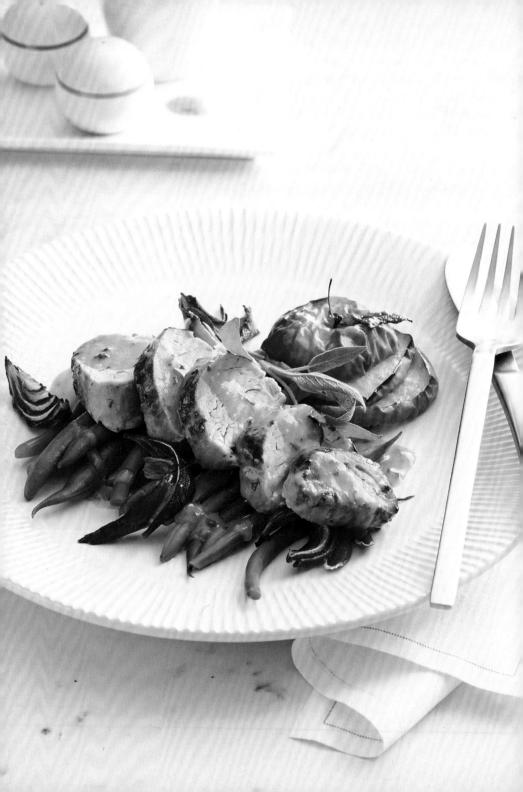

quick roast pork with apple & sage onions

serves 2
prep + cook time 45 minutes
nutritional count per serving 6.7g total fat
(1.3g saturated fat); 1496kJ (358 cal); 38.5g
carbohydrate; 33.4g protein; 6.6g fibre

2 teaspoons olive oil
240g (8oz) lean pork fillet
1 tablespoon dijon mustard
1 tablespoon finely chopped fresh flat-leaf
    parsley
1 tablespoon honey
1 large red apple (200g), unpeeled, cut into
    5mm (¼-inch) rounds
1 large red onion (200g), cut into thin
    wedges
8 sage leaves
1 tablespoon plain flour
250ml (8fl oz) salt-reduced chicken stock
150g (5oz) green beans, trimmed

358
calorie count per serving

1 Preheat oven to 200°C.
2 Heat half the oil in medium
flameproof baking dish on stove
top; cook pork until browned all
over. Remove from heat. Combine
mustard, parsley and honey in small
bowl; brush mustard mixture all over
pork, season.
3 Place apple, onion and sage
around pork in dish; drizzle with
remaining oil. Roast, uncovered,
in oven, about 20 minutes or until
pork is cooked through. Remove
pork, apples, onion and sage from
dish, cover with foil; stand
10 minutes.
4 Meanwhile, place dish over
medium heat on stove top. Add
flour; cook, stirring, until mixture
thickens and bubbles. Gradually
add stock; cook, stirring, until gravy
boils and thickens slightly. Season
to taste.
5 Boil, steam or microwave beans
until tender; drain. Serve sliced pork
with baked apples, onions and sage,
gravy and beans.

pork & ginger stir-fry

serves 2
prep + cook time 45 minutes
nutritional count per serving 5.5g total fat
(1g saturated fat); 1659kJ (397 cal); 35.8g
carbohydrate; 42.9g protein; 14.5g fibre

4cm (1½-inch) piece fresh ginger (20g),
   grated
60ml (2fl oz) teriyaki sauce
240g (8oz) lean pork fillet, sliced thinly
1 teaspoon groundnut oil
1 medium red onion (170g), cut into thin
   wedges
1 medium red pepper (200g), sliced thinly
115g (3½oz) baby corn, halved
1 large carrot (180g), sliced thinly
175g (6oz) tenderstem broccoli, chopped
   coarsely
60ml (2fl oz) water
200g (7oz) mangetout, trimmed

1 Combine ginger, 1 tablespoon of
the sauce and pork in medium bowl.
2 Heat oil in wok; stir-fry pork, in
batches, until browned. Remove
from wok.
3 Add onion, pepper, corn, carrot,
broccoli and the water to wok; stir-fry
until carrot is tender. Return pork to
wok with mangetout and remaining
sauce; stir-fry until vegetables are
tender. Season to taste.

397
calorie count per serving

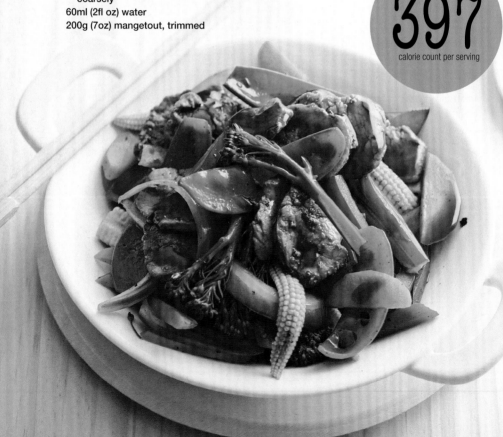

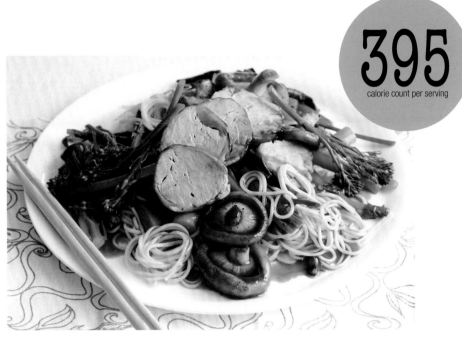

395
calorie count per serving

barbecued pork with noodles

serves 2
prep + cook time 40 minutes
nutritional count per serving 3.8g total fat
(0.8g saturated fat); 1651kJ (395 cal);
35.9g carbohydrate; 43.2g protein; 15.9g fibre

240g (8oz) lean pork fillet, halved
    widthways
2 tablespoons char siu sauce
1 tablespoon water
60g (2oz) dried egg vermicelli
175g (6oz) tenderstem broccoli, chopped
    coarsely
400g (13oz) chinese broccoli, chopped
    coarsely
150g (5oz) fresh shiitake mushrooms
60ml (2fl oz) chicken stock
2 tablespoons oyster sauce
1 tablespoon chinese cooking wine

1 Preheat grill.
2 Cut small slits into both sides
of pork in a criss-cross pattern.
Combine char siu sauce and the
water in shallow dish; add pork, turn
to coat, season.
3 Place pork on wire rack in medium
baking dish; pour enough cold water
into dish until 2cm (¾ inch) deep.
Grill pork about 5 minutes; turn pork,
grill about 5 minutes or until cooked
through. Cover pork; stand 5 minutes
then slice thinly.
4 Meanwhile, place noodles in small
heatproof bowl, cover with boiling
water; separate with fork, drain.
5 Heat oiled wok; stir-fry the broccoli,
mushrooms, stock, oyster sauce and
wine until vegetables are tender. Add
noodles; stir-fry until hot. Season to
taste. Serve noodle stir-fry with pork.

pork rissoles with peppered greens

serves 2
prep + cook time 45 minutes (+ refrigeration)
nutritional count per serving 4g total fat
(1g saturated fat); 1480kJ (354 cal); 18.4g
carbohydrate; 45.1g protein; 10.2g fibre

300g (10oz) lean minced pork
2 cloves garlic, crushed
1 small brown onion (100g), chopped finely
4 tablespoons coarsely chopped fresh mint
1 egg white, beaten lightly
25g (1 oz) stale breadcrumbs
6 medium swiss chard leaves (390g),
    trimmed, shredded coarsely
160g (5½oz) finely shredded savoy
    cabbage
100g (3½oz) baby spinach leaves
½ teaspoon coarse ground black pepper
1½ teaspoons dijon mustard
2 teaspoons plain flour
125ml (4fl oz) chicken stock
125ml (4fl oz) dry white wine

1 Combine pork, half the garlic, and all the onion, mint, egg white and breadcrumbs in medium bowl; season. Shape pork mixture into six patties; place on tray. Cover; refrigerate 30 minutes.
2 Heat large non-stick frying pan over medium heat; cook swiss chard, cabbage, spinach, pepper and remaining garlic, stirring, about 5 minutes or until greens wilt. Season to taste. Remove from pan; cover to keep warm.
3 Cook patties in same pan until browned both sides and cooked through. Remove from pan; cover to keep warm.
4 Add mustard, flour, stock and wine to pan; cook, stirring, until mixture boils and thickens. Strain sauce into small heatproof jug. Serve rissoles with greens and sauce.

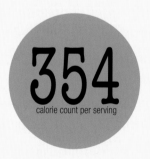

354
calorie count per serving

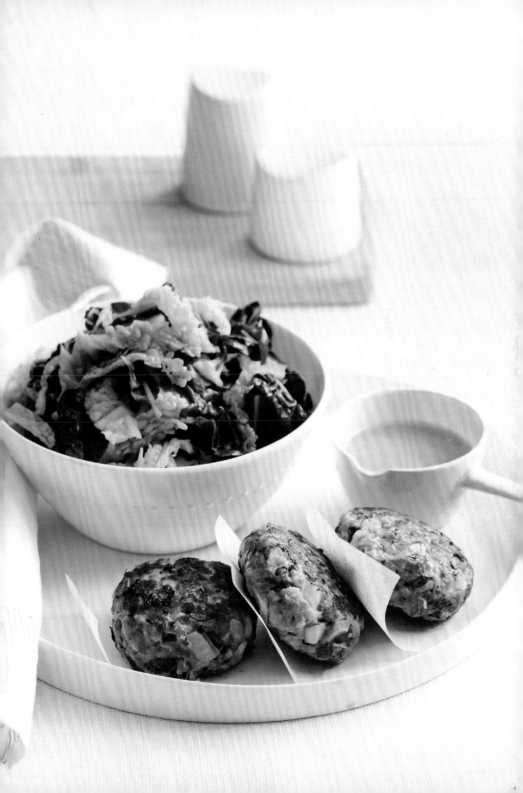

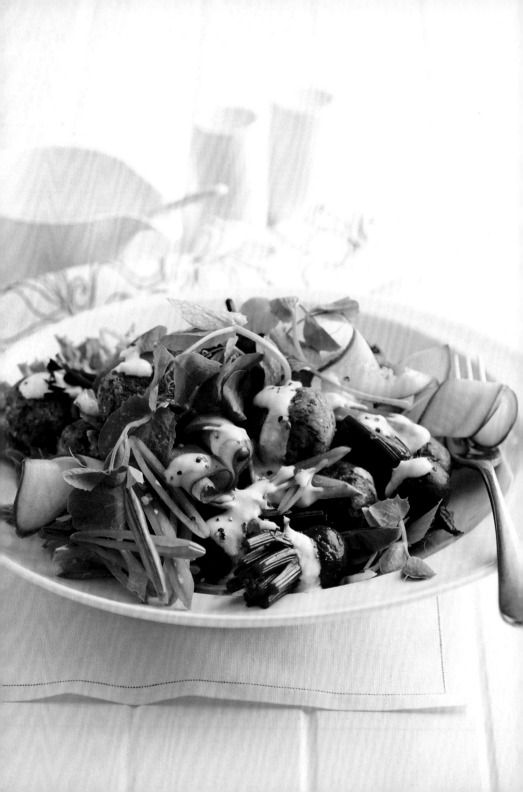

falafel with beetroot & mixed green salad

serves 2
prep + cook time 1 hour (+ refrigeration)
nutritional count per serving 7.8g total fat
(1.1g saturated fat); 1639kJ (392 cal); 51.4g
carbohydrate; 20.5g protein; 18.4g fibre

1 spring onion, chopped finely
1 teaspoon each ground cumin and
   coriander
60g (2oz) frozen peas, thawed
6 tablespoons each fresh coriander and
   mint leaves
250g (8oz) canned chickpeas, rinsed,
   drained
1 egg white
35g stale breadcrumbs
500g (1lb) fresh baby beetroot
60g (2oz) pea shoots
30g (1oz) mixed salad leaves
½ cucumber (130g), cut into ribbons
125g (4oz) sugar snap peas, trimmed,
   sliced thinly
2 teaspoons olive oil

yogurt & garlic dressing
2 tablespoons fat-free natural yogurt
1 tablespoon water
2 teaspoons lemon juice
1 small clove garlic, crushed

1 Blend or process onion, spices, peas, coriander, mint, chickpeas, egg white and breadcrumbs until mixture forms a coarse paste; season. Shape level tablespoons of mixture into balls. Place on baking-parchment-lined tray, cover; refrigerate 30 minutes.
2 Meanwhile, trim beetroot, leaving 2cm (¾ inch) of stem attached. Boil, steam or microwave beetroot until tender; drain. When cool enough to handle, peel beetroot.
3 Combine pea shoots, salad leaves, cucumber, sugar snap peas and beetroot on serving plates.
4 Heat oil in medium frying pan; cook falafel until browned lightly and heated through.
5 Meanwhile, make yogurt and garlic dressing: combine ingredients in small bowl; season to taste.
6 Top salad with falafel and drizzle with dressing.

tips Use a vegetable peeler to slice the cucumber lengthways into thin ribbons. Use disposable gloves when handling beetroot to stop it from staining your hands.

392
calorie count per serving

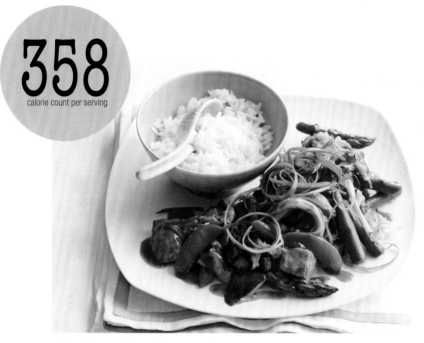

358 calorie count per serving

chilli tofu & mushroom stir-fry

serves 2
prep + cook time 30 minutes
nutritional count per serving 6.3g total fat
(0.7g saturated fat); 1496kJ (358 cal); 44.4g
carbohydrate; 24.3g protein; 12.3g fibre

65g (2½oz) jasmine rice
2 spring onions, sliced thinly lengthways
2 teaspoons cornflour
2 tablespoons water
2 tablespoons japanese soy sauce
2 tablespoons sweet chilli sauce
1 tablespoon chinese cooking wine
100g (3½oz) packaged marinated chilli tofu
　　pieces, chopped coarsely
340g (12oz) asparagus, trimmed, chopped
　　coarsely
100g (3½oz) fresh shiitake mushrooms,
　　halved
200g (7oz) sugar snap peas, trimmed
160g (5½oz) finely shredded chinese
　　cabbage
4cm (1½-inch) piece fresh ginger (20g), cut
　　into matchsticks
100g (3½oz) enoki mushrooms, trimmed

1 Bring medium saucepan of water
to the boil, gradually add rice; boil
uncovered about 20 minutes or until
rice is tender, drain.
2 Place onions in small bowl of iced
water; set aside. Blend cornflour with
the water, sauces and cooking wine
in small jug.
3 Heat lightly oiled wok; stir-fry tofu,
asparagus, shiitake mushrooms
and peas about 5 minutes or until
vegetables soften. Add cabbage,
ginger and enoki mushrooms; stir-fry
until cabbage wilts.
4 Add sauce mixture to wok; stir-fry
until hot. Season to taste. Serve stir-fry
sprinkled with onion; serve with rice.

tip Packaged marinated tofu is
available in the chilled section of
major supermarkets, health-food
shops or from Asian supermarkets.

vegetable biryani

serves 2
prep + cook time 35 minutes
nutritional count per serving 6.4g total fat
(0.6g saturated fat); 1580kJ (378 cal); 62.9g
carbohydrate; 13.1g protein; 6.6g fibre

1 small brown onion (100g), sliced thinly
2 cloves garlic, crushed
2cm (¾-inch) piece fresh ginger (10g),
    grated
1 cinnamon stick
2 cardamom pods, bruised
1 teaspoon ground cumin
1 fresh small red chilli, sliced thinly
130g (4½oz) basmati rice
330ml (12fl oz) vegetable stock
160ml (5½fl oz) water
1 baby cauliflower (125g), cut into florets
100g (3½oz) button mushrooms, halved
125g (4oz) baby green beans, trimmed
3 tablespoons fresh coriander leaves
1 tablespoon flaked almonds, roasted
2 tablespoons fat-free natural yogurt

1 Heat large non-stick saucepan
over medium heat; cook onion,
garlic and ginger, stirring, until onion
softens. Add spices and half the chilli;
cook, stirring, until fragrant.
2 Add rice; stir to coat in spice
mixture. Add stock, water, cauliflower
and mushrooms; bring to the boil.
Reduce heat; simmer, covered, about
15 minutes or until liquid is absorbed.
Remove from heat; stand, covered,
about 10 minutes or until rice is tender.
Discard cinnamon stick.
3 Meanwhile, boil, steam or
microwave beans until tender; drain.
4 Stir beans into rice; season to
taste. Serve biryani sprinkled with
coriander, nuts and remaining chilli;
accompany with yogurt.

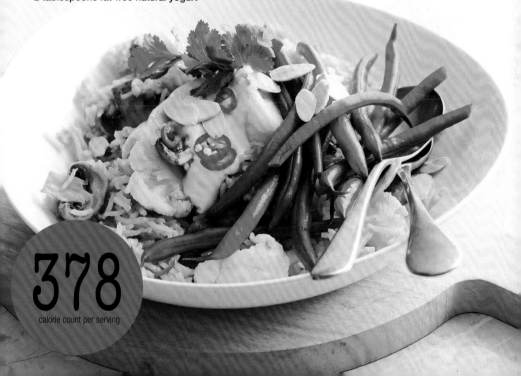

378
calorie count per serving

cauliflower, pumpkin & split pea curry

serves 2
prep + cook time 1 hour
nutritional count per serving 7.5g total fat
(0.9g saturated fat); 1467kJ (351 cal); 39.3g
carbohydrate; 22.8g protein; 14.9g fibre

50g (2oz) yellow split peas
250g (8oz) butternut squash, chopped
  coarsely
1 medium brown onion (170g), chopped
  finely
2 cloves garlic, crushed
2cm (¾-inch) piece fresh ginger (10g),
  grated
1½ tablespoons hot curry paste
375ml (13fl oz) water
250g (8oz) cauliflower, cut into florets
2 large tomatoes (440g), chopped coarsely
60g (2oz) frozen peas
200g (7oz) fat-free natural yogurt
4 tablespoons fresh coriander leaves

1 Cook split peas in medium
saucepan of boiling water about
20 minutes or until almost tender.
Add pumpkin; return to the boil. Boil,
uncovered, about 8 minutes or until
squash is tender; drain.

2 Meanwhile, heat large non-stick
saucepan over medium heat; cook
onion, garlic and ginger, stirring, until
onion softens. Add paste; cook,
stirring, about 2 minutes or until
fragrant.

3 Add the water; bring to the boil.
Reduce heat, add cauliflower and
tomato; simmer, covered, stirring
occasionally, about 10 minutes or
until cauliflower is tender and curry
is thick.

4 Add squash and split pea mixture,
peas and yogurt to curry; stir over low
heat until mixture is heated through.
Season to taste. Serve curry sprinkled
with coriander.

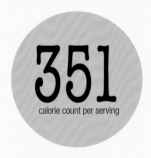

351

calorie count per serving

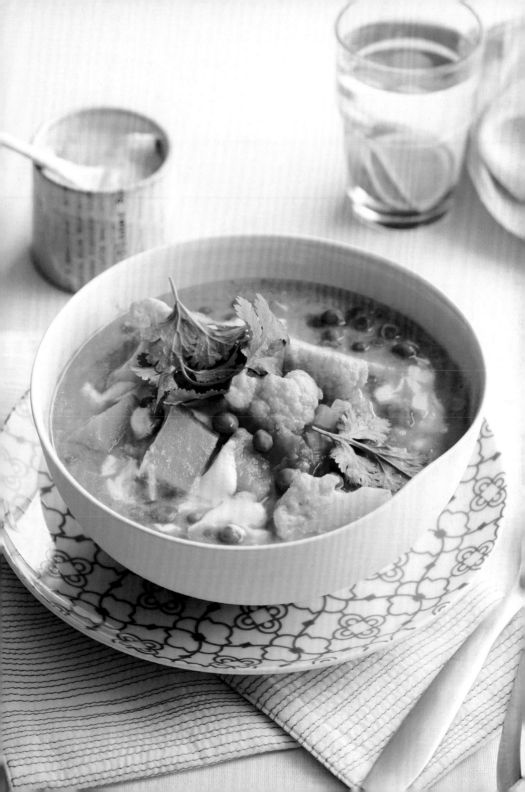

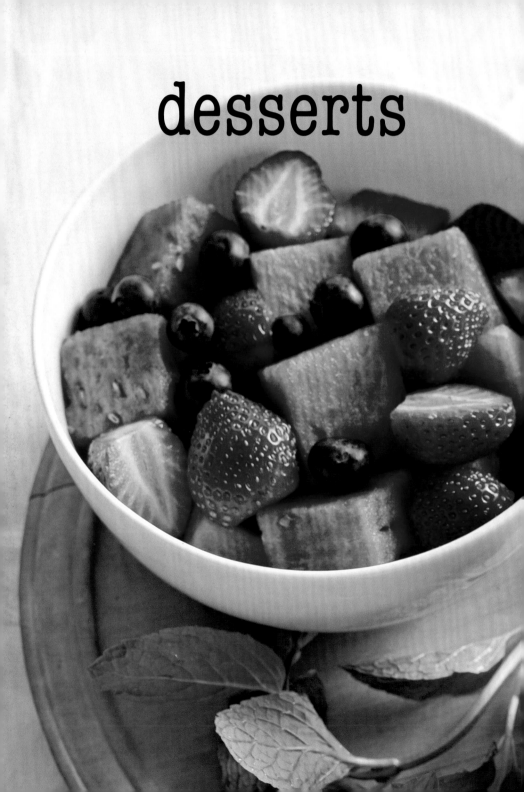

desserts

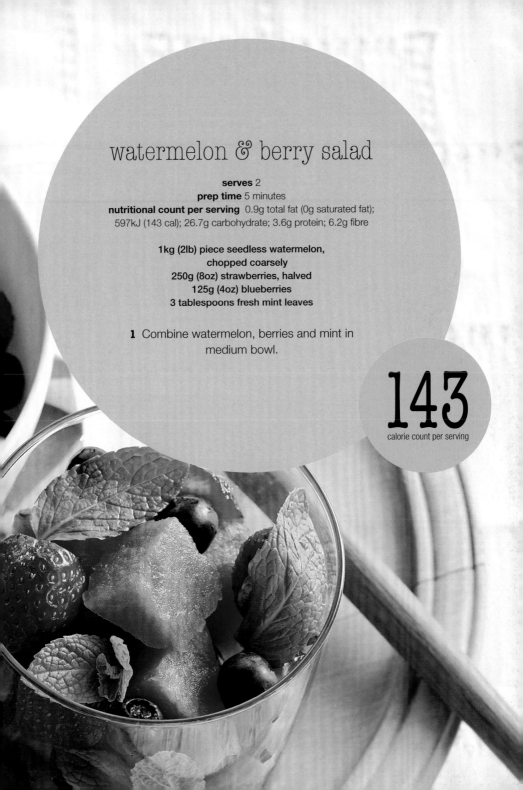

watermelon & berry salad

serves 2
prep time 5 minutes
nutritional count per serving 0.9g total fat (0g saturated fat);
597kJ (143 cal); 26.7g carbohydrate; 3.6g protein; 6.2g fibre

1kg (2lb) piece seedless watermelon,
chopped coarsely
250g (8oz) strawberries, halved
125g (4oz) blueberries
3 tablespoons fresh mint leaves

1 Combine watermelon, berries and mint in
medium bowl.

143
calorie count per serving

vanilla panna cotta with berry compote

serves 2
prep + cook time 40 minutes (+ refrigeration)
nutritional count per serving 7.6g total fat
(4.7g saturated fat); 836kJ (200 cal); 24.5g
carbohydrate; 7.2g protein; 2g fibre

½ vanilla pod
80ml (3floz) reduced fat double cream
1 tablespoon caster sugar
¾ teaspoon gelatine
2 tablespoons boiling water
140g (5oz) fat-free natural yogurt

berry compote
1 cinnamon stick
75g (3oz) frozen or fresh mixed berries
1 tablespoon caster sugar
2 tablespoons boiling water, extra

200
calorie count per serving

1 Scrape seeds from vanilla pod into small saucepan; discard pod. Add cream and sugar to pan; cook, stirring, over low heat, about 5 minutes or until sugar dissolves and mixture is hot.

2 Sprinkle the gelatine over 2 tablespoons boiling water in small heatproof jug; stir until gelatine dissolves. Stir gelatine mixture into cream mixture; cool 5 minutes.

3 Whisk yogurt into cream mixture until smooth. Pour mixture into two 125ml (4floz) moulds, cover loosely with cling film; refrigerate 4 hours or overnight until set.

4 Combine cinnamon stick, berries, sugar and 2 tablespoons boiling water in small bowl; stir until sugar dissolves. Cover; refrigerate until required. Just before serving, turn panna cotta onto serving plates. Discard cinnamon stick from compote; serve compote with panna cotta.

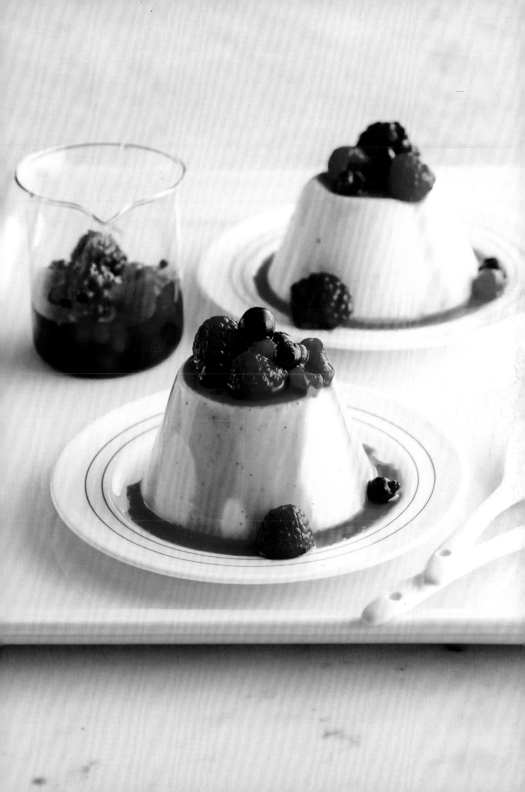

blackberry apple crumbles

serves 2
prep + cook time 50 minutes
nutritional count per serving 3.3g total fat
(0.3g saturated fat); 1066kJ (255 cal); 51.2g
carbohydrate; 3.2g protein; 7g fibre

400g (13oz) canned apples
75g (3oz) frozen blackberries
1 tablespoon caster sugar
30g (1oz) rolled oats
1 tablespoon maple syrup
1 tablespoon flaked almonds
¼ teaspoon ground cinnamon

1 Preheat oven to 180°C. Grease
two 250ml (8floz) ovenproof dishes.
2 Combine apple, blackberries and
sugar in medium bowl; spoon mixture
into dishes.
3 Combine oats, maple syrup,
almonds and cinnamon in small bowl;
sprinkle crumble mixture over fruit
mixture.
4 Bake, uncovered, about 40
minutes or until browned lightly.

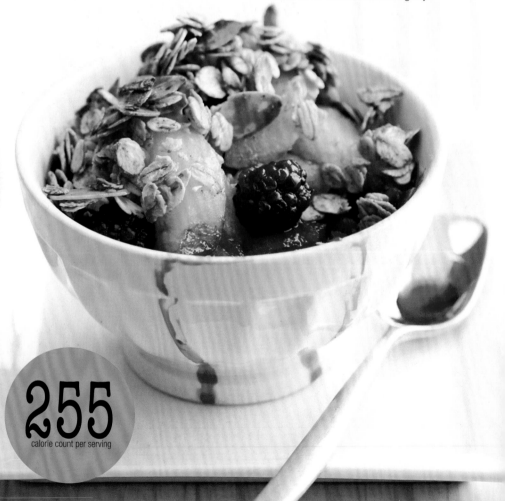

255
calorie count per serving

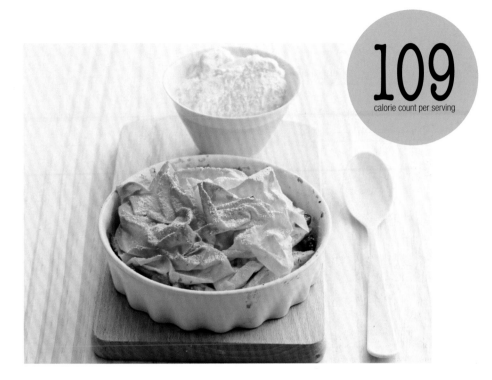

109
calorie count per serving

apple & pear pies

serves 2
prep + cook time 55 minutes
nutritional count per serving 0.7g total fat
(0.2g saturated fat); 458kJ (109 cal); 23.5g
carbohydrate; 1.6g protein; 2.5g fibre

1 medium apple (150g)
1 small pear (180g)
1 tablespoon lemon juice
2 tablespoons finely chopped dried figs
1 tablespoon caster sugar
½ teaspoon ground cinnamon
2 sheets filo pastry
cooking oil spray
2 teaspoons sifted icing sugar
2 heaped tablespoons low-fat ice-cream

1 Preheat oven to 180°C.
2 Peel, core and thinly slice apple
and pear; combine fruit with lemon
juice, figs, sugar and cinnamon in
medium bowl.
3 Divide fruit mixture between
two shallow 250ml (8floz) ovenproof
dishes; cover with foil. Bake about
10 minutes or until fruit starts to
soften.
4 Remove foil; top each dish with a
scrunched sheet of filo pastry. Spray
pastry with cooking oil; bake about
30 minutes or until browned lightly.
5 Dust each with icing sugar; serve
pies with ice-cream.

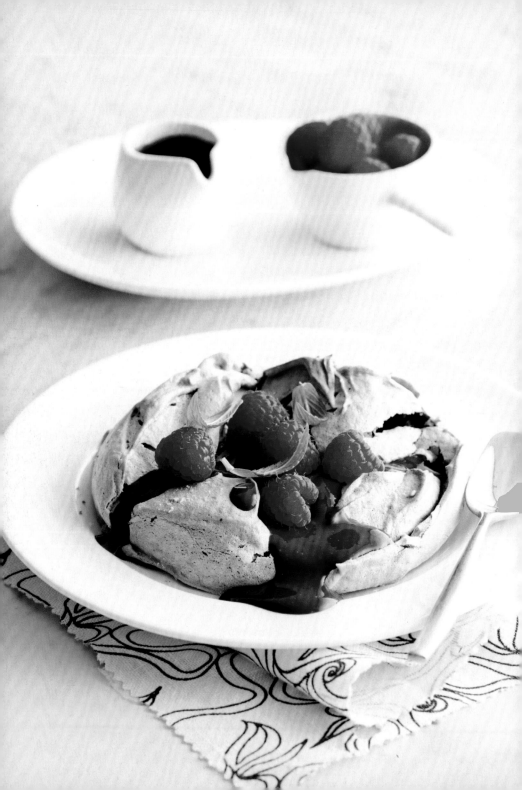

choc-mint mousse pavlovas

serves 2
prep + cook time 50 minutes
nutritional count per serving 1g total fat
(0.5g saturated fat); 811kJ (194 cal); 39g
carbohydrate; 7.4g protein; 2g fibre

2 teaspoons custard powder
1 tablespoon cocoa powder, sifted
2 teaspoons caster sugar
125ml (4floz) skimmed milk
¼ teaspoon peppermint essence
   (or to taste)
60g (2oz) fresh raspberries
1 tablespoon small fresh mint leaves

pavlovas
2 egg whites
75g (3oz) caster sugar
2 teaspoons cocoa powder, sifted

1 Preheat oven to 180°C. Line oven
tray with baking parchment.
2 To make the pavlovas, beat egg
whites in small bowl with electric
mixer until soft peaks form. Gradually
add sugar, one tablespoon at a time,
beating until dissolved. Fold cocoa
powder into meringue mixture. Drop
mixture, in two equal mounds, on
tray. Bake about 25 minutes.
3 Meanwhile, blend custard powder,
cocoa powder and sugar with milk in
small saucepan; cook, stirring, until
sauce boils and thickens. Remove
from heat; stir in peppermint essence.
4 Serve warm pavlovas topped with
sauce, raspberries and mint leaves.

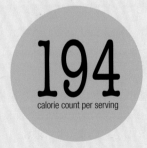

194
calorie count per serving

mango & passionfruit pops

makes 10
prep + cook time 15 minutes (+ freezing)
nutritional count per serving 2.9g total fat
(1.8g saturated fat); 443kJ (106 cal); 16.8g
carbohydrate; 2.6g protein; 2g fibre

2 small mangoes (600g)
60ml (2floz) passionfruit pulp
2 tablespoons icing sugar
50g (2oz) white eating chocolate, coarsely
    grated
375ml (13floz) low-fat vanilla ice-cream,
    softened

1 Peel and coarsely chop mangoes; blend or process mango until pureed (you need about 250m/8floz purée).

2 Combine purée, passionfruit pulp, icing sugar, chocolate and ice-cream in medium bowl.

3 Divide mango mixture into 10 x 60ml (2floz) ice-lolly moulds. Replace lids on moulds and insert lollipop sticks. Freeze 6 hours or overnight.

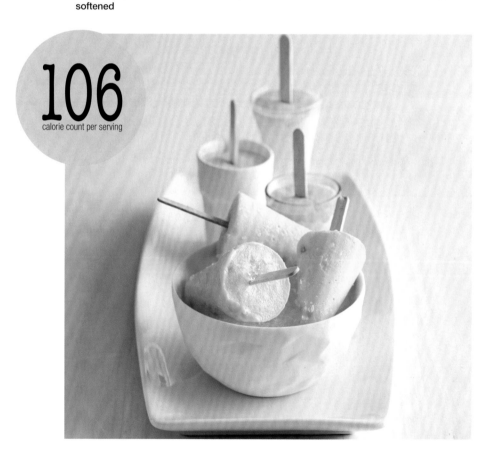

106
calorie count per serving

fruity coconut rice

serves 2
prep + cook time 30 minutes (+ refrigeration)
nutritional count per serving 4.9g total fat
(4.1g saturated fat); 1049kJ (251 cal); 41.8g
carbohydrate; 6g protein; 6.7g fibre

50g (2oz) arborio rice
70g (2½oz) fat-free natural yogurt
125ml (4floz) light coconut milk
1 tablespoon caster sugar
1 thinly sliced small banana (130g)
2 tablespoons passionfruit pulp

1 Gradually stir rice into medium
saucepan of boiling water; boil,
uncovered, stirring, about 10 minutes
or until rice is tender. Drain.
2 Combine rice, yogurt, coconut milk
and sugar in medium bowl, cover;
refrigerate 3 hours.
3 Divide mixture into bowls; top with
banana and passionfruit pulp.

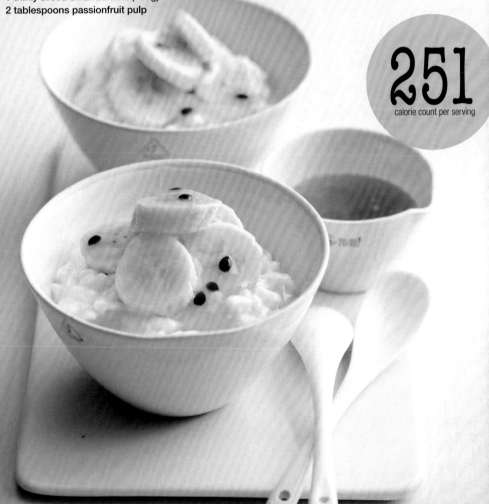

251
calorie count per serving

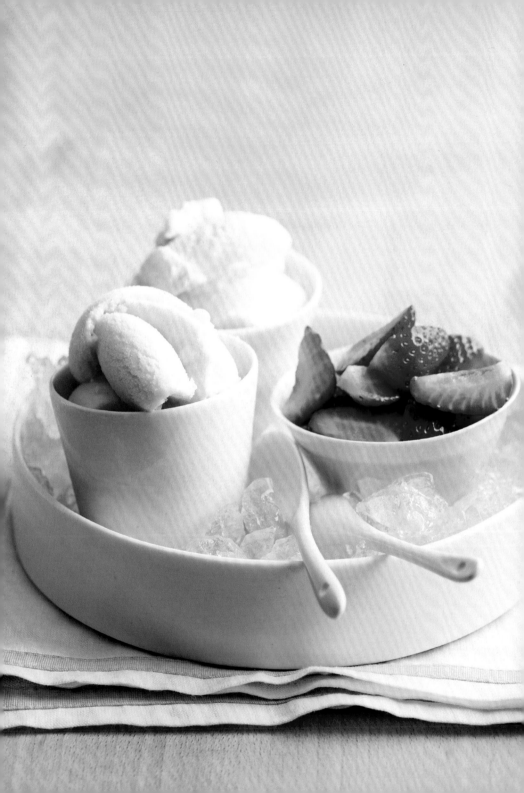

frozen vanilla yogurt

makes 750ml (1½ pints)
prep time 30 minutes (+ freezing) **nutritional count per 200g serving** 0.3g total fat (0.1g saturated fat); 648kJ (155 cal); 25.8g carbohydrate; 11.7g protein; 0g fibre

nutritional count per 200g serving with ½ chopped medium peach 0.3g total fat (0.1g saturated fat); 677kJ (162 cal); 27g carbohydrate; 11.9g protein; 0.3g fibre

nutritional count per 200g serving with 125g strawberries 0.3g total fat (0.1g saturated fat); 740kJ (177 cal); 28.3g carbohydrate; 12.7g protein; 2.8g fibre

2 teaspoons gelatine
2 tablespoons boiling water
90g (3oz) honey
500g (1lb) fat-free natural yogurt
2 egg whites
1 tablespoon vanilla extract
½ medium peach (60g), chopped or
  125g (4oz) strawberries, quartered

1 Sprinkle gelatine over boiling water in small heatproof jug; stir until gelatine dissolves. Cool 5 minutes.
2 Combine honey and yogurt in medium bowl; stir in gelatine mixture. Pour into shallow freezer-proof container, cover with foil; freeze about 2 hours or until set.
3 Process frozen yogurt mixture with egg whites and vanilla extract until smooth. Return to container, cover; freeze yogurt 3 hours or overnight until set.
4 Serve yogurt with chopped peach or strawberries.

tip Frozen yogurt can be made up to 3 days ahead; keep tightly covered with foil in the freezer.

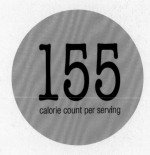

155 calorie count per serving

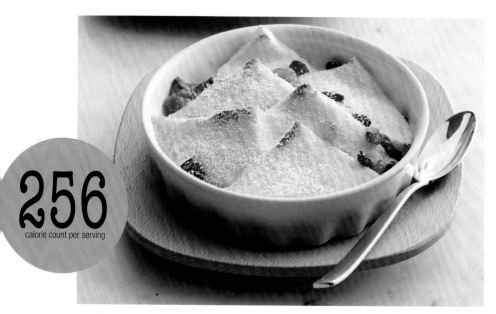

sultana & apricot custard pudding

serves 2
prep + cook time 40 minutes (+ standing)
nutritional count per serving 3.7g total fat
(1g saturated fat); 1070kJ (256 cal); 45.6g
carbohydrate; 10.2g protein; 1.9g fibre

3 slices white bread
1 tablespoon sultanas
1 tablespoon finely chopped dried
   apricots
1 teaspoon icing sugar, sifted

custard
180ml (6½floz) skimmed milk
1 teaspoon vanilla extract
1 egg
2 tablespoons caster sugar

1 Preheat oven to 180°C. Grease
two 180ml (6½floz) ovenproof
dishes.

2 Remove crusts from bread; cut
each slice into quarters. Layer bread,
overlapping slightly, sultanas and
apricots in dishes.

3 To make custard: bring milk and
extract to the boil in small saucepan.
Whisk egg and sugar in small bowl
until combined. Gradually whisk hot
milk mixture into egg mixture.

4 Pour custard over bread; stand
15 minutes.

5 Place dishes in small baking dish.
Pour enough boiling water into baking
dish to come halfway up sides of
dishes. Bake about 25 minutes or
until puddings set. Remove puddings
from dish; stand 5 minutes before
dusting with icing sugar to serve.

crêpes with roasted strawberries

serves 2
prep + cook time 20 minutes
nutritional count per serving 0.4g total fat
(0g saturated fat); 669kJ (160 cal); 31.2g
carbohydrate; 5.2g protein; 5g fibre

250g (8oz) strawberries, halved
1 tablespoon caster sugar
½ teaspoon vanilla extract
1 small orange (180g)
35g (1½oz) plainflour
1 tablespoon skimmed milk
80ml (3floz) water
1 tablespoon finely shredded fresh mint

1 Preheat oven to 180°C. Line shallow baking dish with baking parchment.
2 Place strawberries in dish; sprinkle with sugar, drizzle with vanilla extract, turn gently to combine. Roast, uncovered, about 7 minutes or until strawberries start to soften.
3 Segment orange. Remove dish from oven; stir in orange segments.
4 Meanwhile, sift flour into small bowl; gradually whisk in milk combined with water, until batter is smooth.
5 Heat non-stick frying pan over medium heat; pour in half the batter, tilt pan to cover base. Cook crêpe until browned lightly, loosening edge with spatula. Turn crêpe; brown other side. Remove from pan; cover to keep warm. Repeat with remaining batter.
6 Serve crêpe topped with strawberry mixture and mint.

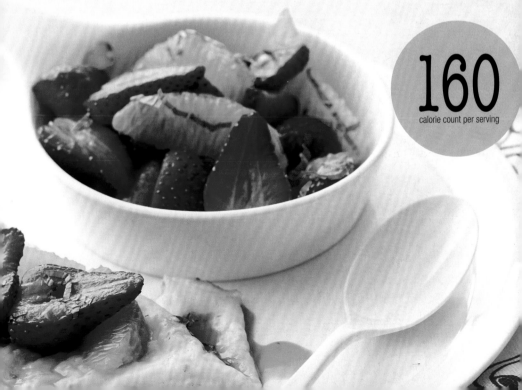

160
calorie count per serving

blueberry trifles

serves 2
prep + cook time 20 minutes (+ refrigeration)
nutritional count per serving 2.8g total fat
(1.4g saturated fat); 1049kJ (251 cal); 44.3g
carbohydrate; 10.4g protein; 1.7g fibre

½ teaspoon vanilla extract
1 tablespoon icing sugar
210g (7½oz) fat-free natural yogurt
2 jam mini rolls
2 tablespoons orange juice
120g (4oz) blueberries
2 teaspoons finely grated orange rind

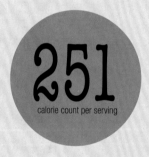

251
calorie count per serving

1 Combine vanilla extract, sugar and
yogurt in small bowl.
2 Thinly slice jam mini rolls. Divide
mini roll slices between two 180ml
(6½floz) glasses; drizzle each equally
with orange juice.
3 Top equally with 60g (2oz) of the
blueberries, then with equal amounts
of the yogurt mixture. Refrigerate
about 30 minutes or until cold.
4 Sprinkle equally with remaining
blueberries and orange rind just
before serving.

tips Grate the rind from the orange
before juicing. Trifles can be made a
day ahead and kept, covered, in the
refrigerator. The trifles can be eaten
as soon as they are made, but they
are at their best when served chilled.

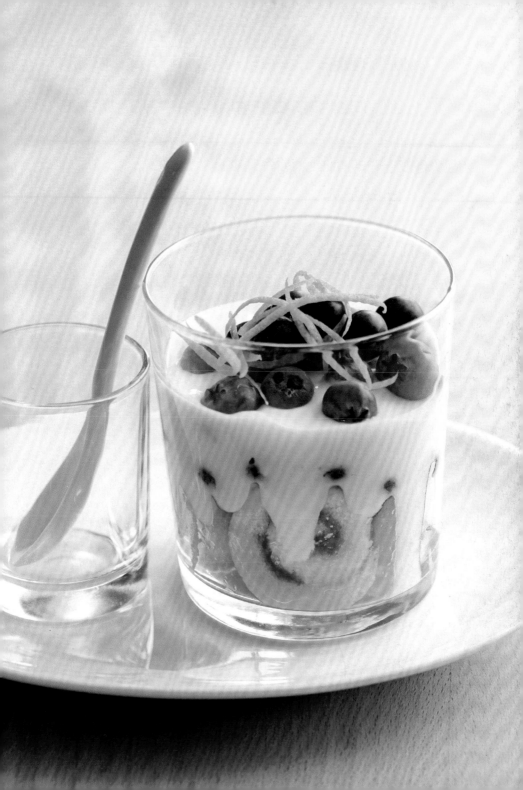

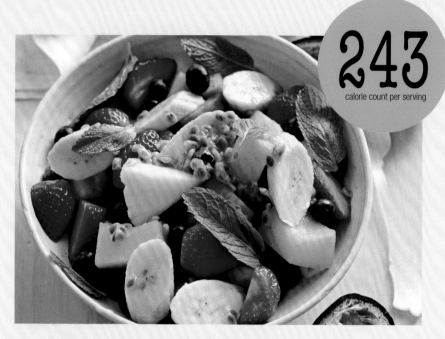

243 calorie count per serving

fruit salad with honey yogurt

serves 2
prep time 15 minutes
nutritional count per serving 0.5g total fat
(0g saturated fat); 1019kJ (243 cal); 47.3g
carbohydrate; 8.1g protein; 7.6g fibre

140g (5oz) fat-free natural yogurt
1 tablespoon honey
100g (3½oz) pineapple, peeled, coarsely
   chopped
100g (3½oz) cantaloupe melon, peeled
   deseeded, coarsely chopped
125g (4oz) strawberries, halved
125g (4oz) blueberries
1 medium banana (200g), sliced thinly
1 tablespoon passionfruit pulp
1 teaspoon lime juice
6 fresh mint leaves

1 Combine yogurt and honey in
small bowl.
2 Just before serving, combine
remaining ingredients in large bowl;
serve with honey yogurt.

tips You only need small quantities
of the pineapple and melon for this
recipe, so buy the smallest ones you
can find. Two passionfruit will supply
the right amount of pulp. Lime juice
not only adds flavour to this recipe,
but also prevents the banana from
discolouring. Honey yogurt can be
made a day ahead; store, covered,
in the refrigerator.

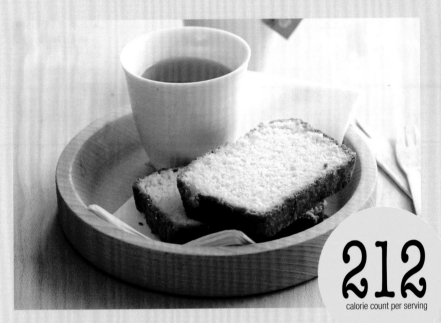

lemony yogurt loaf

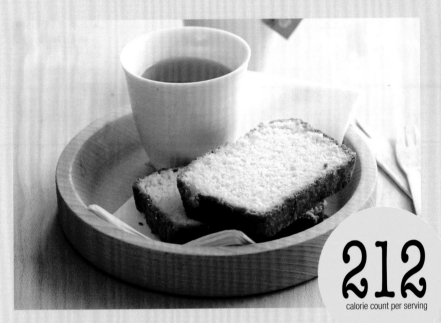
212
calorie count per serving

serves 10
prep + cook time 1½ hours
nutritional count per slice 7.1g total fat
(2.9g saturated fat); 886kJ (212 cal); 50.4g
carbohydrate; 7.4g protein; 1.5g fibre

125g (4oz) reduced-fat olive oil spread
220g (7½oz) caster sugar
2 egg yolks
1½ tablespoons finely grated lemon rind
375g (12oz) self-raising flour, sifted
280g (10oz) fat-free natural yogurt
60ml (2oz) skimmed milk
2 egg whites

1 Preheat oven to 180°C. Grease
14cm x 21cm (5½ inch x 8½-inch)
loaf tin; line base and sides with
baking parchment, extending paper
5cm (2 inches) over sides.

2 Beat olive oil spread, sugar, egg
yolks and lemon rind in small bowl
with electric mixer until changed to a
paler colour. Transfer mixture to large
bowl; stir inflour, yogurt and milk.
3 Beat egg whites in small bowl with
electric mixer until soft peaks form.
Fold about a quarter of the egg white
mixture into lemon mixture, then
gently fold in remaining egg white
mixture.
4 Spread mixture into tin; bake
45 minutes. Reduce oven
temperature to 160°C; bake about
25 minutes. Stand loaf in tin
10 minutes before transferring to
wire rack to cool.

minted fruit salad

serves 2
prep + cook time 35 minutes (+ refrigeration)
nutritional count per serving 0.7g total fat
(0.1g saturated fat); 742kJ (177 cal); 36.1g
carbohydrate; 3.2g protein; 6.4g fibre

180ml (6½floz) water
2 teaspoons grated palm sugar
1 star anise
1 tablespoon lime juice
½ small pineapple (400g), peeled,
    chopped coarsely
½ small honeydew melon (450g), peeled,
    chopped coarsely
250g (8oz) fresh lychees, peeled, seeded
100g (3½oz) seedless red grapes, halved
3 tablespoons fresh mint leaves

1 Stir the water, sugar and star
anise in small saucepan over medium
heat until sugar dissolves. Simmer,
uncovered, 10 minutes. Stir in juice.
Cover; refrigerate 3 hours. Strain
syrup into medium jug; discard
star anise.
2 Combine fruit, mint and syrup in
large bowl.

tips Make syrup the night before.

177
calorie count per serving

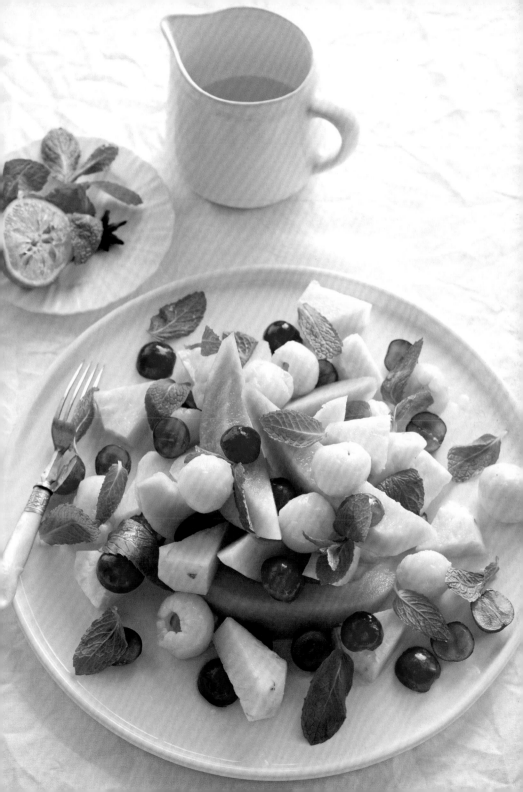

chocolate fudge cakes

makes 10
prep + cook time 35 minutes
nutritional count per cake 6.1g total fat
(3g saturated fat); 895kJ (214cal); 36.1g
carbohydrate; 4.5g protein; 1.1g fibre

50g (2oz) cocoa powder, sifted
165g (6oz) light brown sugar
125ml (4floz) boiling water
75g (3oz) dark eating chocolate, finely
   chopped
2 egg yolks
25g (1oz) ground hazelnuts
50g (2oz) plainflour
4 egg whites

syrup
110g (4oz) light brown sugar
125ml (4floz) water
2 teaspoons instant coffee granules
1 teaspoon sifted cocoa powder

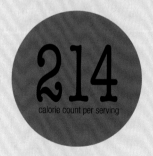

214
calorie count per serving

1 Preheat oven to 170°C. Grease
10-holes of a 12-hole (80ml /3floz)
muffin tin.
2 Combine cocoa powder and sugar
in large bowl; blend in boiling water,
then chocolate, stirring until smooth.
Stir in egg yolks, ground hazelnuts
and flour.
3 Beat egg whites in small bowl
with electric mixer until soft peaks
form. Fold egg whites into chocolate
mixture, in two batches; divide
mixture into holes of muffin tin. Bake
about 15 minutes.
4 Meanwhile, to make syrup, stir
sugar and water in small saucepan
over low heat until sugar dissolves;
bring to the boil. Reduce heat;
simmer, uncovered, without stirring,
about 10 minutes or until syrup
thickens. Stir in coffee granules and
cocoa powder; strain into small
heatproof jug.
5 Stand cakes in tin 5 minutes
before serving warm, drizzled with
syrup.

tip The cakes can be frozen for
ready-made treats. Thaw at room
temperature as required.

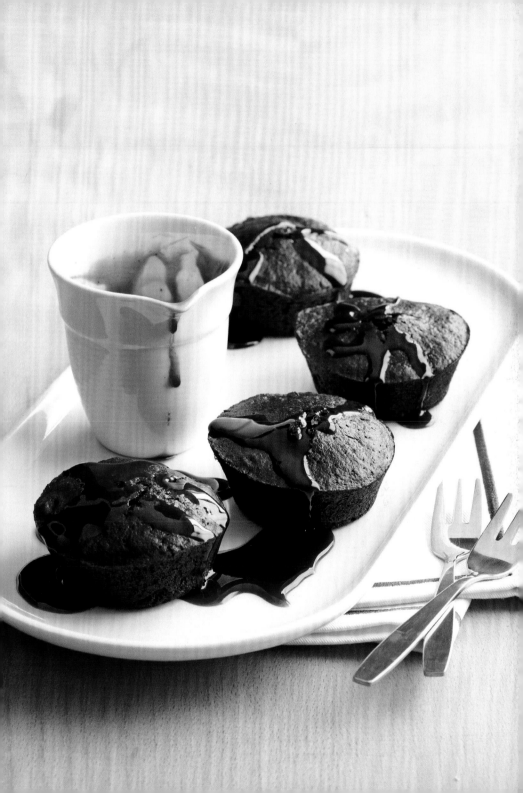

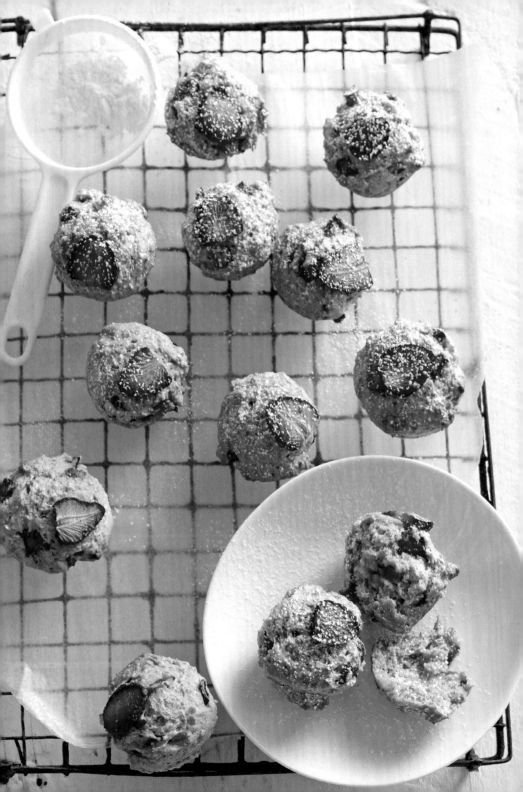

strawberry & rhubarb muffins

makes 24
prep + cook time 35 minutes
nutritional count per muffin 1.2g total fat
(0.2g saturated fat); 233kJ (56 cal); 9g
carbohydrate; 1.7g protein; 1.3g fibre

30g (1oz) low-fat margarine
240g (8½oz) wholemeal self-raising flour
55g (2oz) brown sugar
½ teaspoon ground cinnamon
½ teaspoon vanilla extract
80ml (3floz) skimmed milk
1 egg, beaten lightly
60g (2oz) small strawberries
55g (2oz) finely chopped rhubarb
1½ tablespoons apple sauce

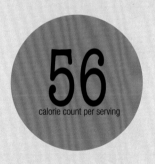

56
calorie count per serving

1 Preheat oven to 180°C. Grease
24-hole mini muffin tin (20ml/2floz).
2 Melt margarine; cool slightly.
Combine flour, sugar and cinnamon
in large bowl. Add vanilla, margarine,
milk and egg; mix to combine.
3 Slice strawberries thinly. Reserve
24 slices. Chop remaining slices
finely; gently stir into batter with the
rhubarb and apple sauce.
4 Spoon mixture into muffin tin; top
each muffin with a strawberry slice.
Bake about 15 minutes.

tips You need about two large
trimmed rhubarb stems for this
recipe. Muffins can be served warm
or at room temperature.

index

antipasto, baked ricotta 61
apple
    apple & pear pies 121
    blackberry apple crumbles 120
    blueberry & apple bircher
        muesli 19
    quick roast pork with apple &
        sage onions 105
apricot
    apricot & coconut muesli 15
    sultana & apricot custard
        pudding 128
asparagus: caesar salad with
    baked asparagus 46
aubergine dip, garlicky 37

banana
    banana, mango & raspberry
        smoothie 18
    crêpes with banana &
        passionfruit syrup 20
    fruity coconut rice 125
    rice flake porridge with banana
        16
barbecued pork with noodles 107
barley risotto with chicken, leek &
    peas 79
beef
    beef & lentil lasagne 101
    beef with black bean sauce 98
    beef with red wine sauce &
        sweet potato crush 103
    vietnamese beef pho 102
beetroot
    english muffin with beetroot
        juice 25
    felafel with beetroot & mixed
        green salad 111
berries (mixed)
    berry & lime fruit salad 39
    oat porridge with berry
        compote 17
    vanilla panna cotta with berry
        compote 118
    watermelon & berry salad 117
bircher muesli, blueberry & apple
    19
biryani, vegetable 113
blackberry apple crumbles 120
blueberry
    berry & lime fruit salad 39
    blueberry & apple bircher
        muesli 19
    blueberry trifles 130
    watermelon & berry salad 117
bread (see also english muffins;
    tortillas; rolls, wraps)
    grilled vegetables with ricotta 28
    panzanella 57
    rye toasts with roasted tomato
        & basil 29
    salmon bruschetta 72
    tuna sushi sandwiches 45
bruschetta, salmon 72
burger, courgette 69
cacciatore, chicken 77
caesar salad with baked
    asparagus 46

cakes (see also muffins)
    chocolate fudge cakes 138
    lemony yogurt loaf 137
cauliflower, pumpkin & split pea
    curry 114
chermoulla lamb with chickpea
    salad 92
cherry parfait 22
chicken
    barley risotto with chicken, leek
        & peas 79
    chicken & corn soup 41
    chicken & soba noodle salad 53
    chicken cacciatore 77
    chicken tabbouleh 64
    mexican chicken wrap 44
    nam jim chicken with rice
        noodle salad 81
    sweet chilli chicken stir-fry 78
    teriyaki chicken rice salad 56
    warm indian-style chicken salad
        54
chickpeas
    chermoulla lamb with chickpea
        salad 92
    chickpea & cumin dip 36
chilli jam lamb with char-grilled
    vegetables 70
chilli tofu & mushroom stir-fry 112
choc-mint mousse pavlovas 123
chocolate fudge cakes 136
cinnamon crisps 35
coconut
    apricot & coconut muesli 15
    fruity coconut rice 125
coleslaw: ham & basil coleslaw
    rolls 44
corn: chicken & corn soup 41
courgette
    courgette burger 69
    lamb cutlets with parsnip mash
        & courgette salad 95
couscous: moroccan fish kebabs
    with couscous salad 82
crêpes
    with banana & passionfruit
        syrup 20
    with roasted strawberries 129
crisps
    cinnamon 35
    seeded mustard 35
crumbles, blackberry apple 120
curry, cauliflower, pumpkin & split
    pea 114

dips
    chickpea & cumin 36
    garlicky aubergine 37

eggs
    ham, egg & vegetable fried rice
        65
    mexican-style tortilla 75
    mixed mushroom & herb
        omelette 32
    primavera frittata 62
english muffin
    with beetroot juice 25
    with mint & pineapple juice 24

falafel with beetroot & mixed green
    salad 111
fish (see also salmon; tuna)
    baked fish fillets with chilli
        potatoes 87
    kerala-style fish with lime pickle
        yogurt 85
    moroccan fish kebabs with
        couscous salad 82
    thai-style fish cakes with
        cucumber chilli pickle 88
five-spice lamb and chilli stir-fry
    with greens 94
frappé, melon & raspberry 38
frittata, primavera 62
frozen vanilla yogurt 127
fruit (dried)
    fruit nibble mix 34
    sultana & apricot custard
        pudding 128
fruit salads
    berry & lime 39
    minted 134
    papaya & orange 21
    watermelon & berry 117
    with honey yogurt 132
fruity coconut rice 125

garlicky aubergine dip 37
ginger: pork & ginger stir-fry 106
grape: raspberry & grape jelly 39
greens
    five-spice lamb and chilli stir-fry
        with greens 94
    pork rissoles with peppered
        greens 108

ham
    ham & basil coleslaw rolls 44
    ham, egg & vegetable fried rice
        65
    ham salad lettuce wraps 36
    vegetable rösti with ham &
        roasted tomatoes 30
honey
    fruit salad with honey yogurt
        133
    honey spiced salmon with nashi
        pear salad 91
    pancakes with honey pears 27
hot & sour vegetable soup 43
hummus, sweet potato with
    vegetables 60

jelly, raspberry & grape 39
juice
    beetroot 25
    mint & pineapple 24

kebabs: moroccan fish kebabs
    with couscous salad 82
kerala-style fish with lime pickle
    yogurt 85

lamb
    chermoulla lamb with chickpea
        salad 92
    chilli jam lamb with char-grilled
        vegetables 70
    five-spice lamb and chilli stir-fry
        with greens 94

grilled pepper lamb with roast vegetables 97
lamb cutlets with parsnip mash & courgette salad 95
spiced lamb cutlets with tomato parsley salad 68
lasagne, beef & lentil 101
lassi, pineapple & strawberry 38
leek: barley risotto with chicken, leek & peas 79
lemony yogurt loaf 133
lentils
 beef & lentil lasagne 101
 spiced red lentil soup 42
 spicy vegetable & lentil salad 51
lime: berry & lime fruit salad 39
mango
 banana, mango & raspberry smoothie 18
 mango & passionfruit pops 124
melon
 melon & raspberry frappé 38
 watermelon & berry salad 117
mexican chicken wrap 44
mexican-style tortilla 75
mint
 choc-mint mousse pavlovas 123
 english muffin with mint & pineapple juice 24
 minted fruit salad 134
 mint sauce 70
moroccan fish kebabs with couscous salad 82
muesli
 apricot & coconut 15
 blueberry & apple bircher 19
muffins, strawberry & rhubarb 141
mushrooms
 chilli tofu & mushroom stir-fry 112
 mixed mushroom & herb omelette 32

nam jim chicken with rice noodle salad 81
nashi pear salad 91
niçoise salad 52
noodles
 barbecued pork with noodles 107
 chicken & soba noodle salad 53
 hot & sour vegetable soup 43
 nam jim chicken with rice noodle salad 81
 prawn & rice vermicelli salad 49
 szechuan-style prawns with rice noodles 84

oat porridge with berry compote 17
omelette, mixed mushroom & herb 32
onions: quick roast pork with apple & sage onions 105
orange: papaya & orange salad 21

pancakes with honey pears 27
panna cotta, vanilla with berry compote 118
panzanella 57

papaya & orange salad 21
pappardelle with fresh tomato sauce 73
parfait, cherry 22
parsnip: lamb cutlets with parsnip mash & courgette salad 95
passionfruit
 crêpes with banana & passionfruit syrup 20
 mango & passionfruit pops 124
pasta
 pappardelle with fresh tomato sauce 73
 tuna macaroni salad 50
pavlovas, choc-mint mousse 123
pears
 apple & pear pies 121
 honey spiced salmon with nashi pear salad 91
 pancakes with honey pears 27
peas
 barley risotto with chicken, leek & peas 79
 cauliflower, pumpkin & split pea curry 114
pies, apple & pear 121
pineapple
 english muffin with mint & pineapple juice 24
 pineapple & strawberry lassi 38
pizza: potato & rosemary pizza with garden salad 67
popcorn, spiced 34
pops, mango & passionfruit 124
pork
 barbecued pork with noodles 107
 pork & ginger stir-fry 106
 pork rissoles with peppered greens 108
 quick roast pork with apple & sage onions 105
porridge
 oat with berry compote 17
 rice flake with banana 16
potatoes
 baked fish fillets with chilli potatoes 87
 lamb cutlets with parsnip mash & courgette salad 95
 potato & rosemary pizza with garden salad 67
 primavera frittata 62
prawns
 prawn & rice vermicelli salad 49
 szechuan-style prawns with rice noodles 84
primavera frittata 62
pudding, sultana & apricot custard 128
pumpkin: cauliflower, pumpkin & split pea curry 114

raspberry
 banana, mango & raspberry smoothie 18
 melon & raspberry frappé 38
 raspberry & grape jelly 39
rhubarb: strawberry & rhubarb muffins 141

rice
 barley risotto with chicken, leek & peas 79
 fruity coconut rice 125
 ham, egg & vegetable fried rice 65
 rice flake porridge with banana 16
 teriyaki chicken rice salad 56
ricotta
 baked ricotta antipasto 61
 grilled vegetables with ricotta 28
rissoles, pork with peppered greens 108
risotto, barley with chicken, leek & peas 79
rolls
 ham & basil coleslaw 44
 shredded vegetable rice paper 58
 vietnamese-style vegetable 45
rösti, vegetable with ham & roasted tomatoes 30
rye toasts with roasted tomato & basil 29

salads (see also fruit salads)
 caesar salad with baked asparagus 46
 chicken & soba noodle 53
 chickpea 92
 courgette 95
 couscous 82
 garden 67
 ham salad lettuce wraps 36
 mixed green 111
 nashi pear 91
 niçoise 52
 panzanella 57
 prawn & rice vermicelli 49
 rice noodle 81
 spicy vegetable & lentil 51
 teriyaki chicken rice 56
 thai salad cups 37
 tomato parsley 68
 tuna macaroni 50
 tuna waldorf 47
 warm indian-style chicken 54
salmon
 honey spiced salmon with nashi pear salad 91
 salmon bruschetta 72
salsa
 chunky mexican-style 31
 tomato & caper 87
sandwiches, tuna sushi 45
seeded mustard crisps 35
shredded vegetable rice paper rolls 58
smoothie, banana, mango & raspberry 18
soups
 chicken & corn 41
 hot & sour vegetable 43
 spiced red lentil 42
spiced lamb cutlets with tomato parsley salad 68
spiced popcorn 34
spiced red lentil soup 42
spicy vegetable & lentil salad 51

stir-fries
chilli tofu & mushroom 112
five-spice lamb and chilli with
greens 94
pork & ginger 106
sweet chilli chicken 78
strawberry
berry & lime fruit salad 39
crêpes with roasted
strawberries 129
pineapple & strawberry lassi 38
strawberry & rhubarb muffins
138
watermelon & berry salad 117
sultana & apricot custard pudding
128
sweet chilli chicken stir-fry 78
sweet potato
beef with red wine sauce &
sweet potato crush 103
sweet potato hummus with
vegetables 60
szechuan-style prawns with rice
noodles 84

tabbouleh, chicken 64
teriyaki chicken rice salad 56
thai salad cups 37
thai-style fish cakes with
cucumber chilli pickle 88
tofu: chilli tofu & mushroom stir-fry
112

tomatoes
pappardelle with fresh tomato
sauce 73
rye toasts with roasted tomato
& basil 29
spiced lamb cutlets with
tomato parsley salad 68
tomato & caper salsa 87
vegetable rösti with ham &
roasted tomatoes 30
tortilla, mexican-style 75
tortillas: chunky mexican-style
salsa with tortillas 31
trifles, blueberry 130
tuna
niçoise salad 52
tuna macaroni salad 50
tuna sushi sandwiches 45
tuna waldorf salad 47
vanilla
frozen vanilla yogurt 127
vanilla panna cotta with berry
compote 118
vegetables (mixed)
chilli jam lamb with char-grilled
vegetables 70
grilled pepper lamb with roast
vegetables 97
grilled vegetables with ricotta 28
ham, egg & vegetable fried rice
65
hot & sour vegetable soup 43

shredded vegetable rice paper
rolls 58
spicy vegetable & lentil salad 51
sweet potato hummus with
vegetables 60
vegetable biryani 113
vegetable rösti with ham &
roasted tomatoes 30
vietnamese-style vegetable roll
45
vietnamese beef pho 102
vietnamese-style vegetable roll 45

waldorf salad, tuna 47
watermelon & berry salad 117
wraps
ham salad lettuce 36
mexican chicken 44

yogurt
frozen vanilla yogurt 127
fruit salad with honey yogurt
133
kerala-style fish with lime pickle
yogurt 85

conversion charts

WEIGHTS

5g	¼oz
15g	½oz
20g	¾oz
25g	1oz
50g	2oz
65g	2½oz
75g	3oz
125g	4oz
150g	5oz
175g	6oz
200g	7oz
250g	8oz
275g	9oz
300g	10oz
325g	11oz
375g	12oz
400g	13oz
425g	14oz
450g	14½oz
475g	15oz
500g	1lb
625g	1¼lb
750g	1½lb
875g	1¾lb
1kg	2lb

1.25kg	2½lb
1.5 kg	3lb
1.75 kg	3½lb
2 kg	4lb

MEASUREMENTS

2.5mm	⅛ inch
5mm	¼ inch
1cm	½ inch
1.5cm	¾ inch
2.5cm	1 inch
3.5cm	1½ inches
5cm	2 inches
6cm	2½ inches
7cm	3 inches
10cm	4 inches
12cm	5 inches
15cm	6 inches
18cm	7 inches
20cm	8 inches
23cm	9 inches
25cm	10 inches
28cm	11 inches
30cm	12 inches

LIQUIDS

15ml	½fl oz
25ml	1fl oz
50ml	2fl oz
75ml	3fl oz
10ml	3½fl oz
125ml	4fl oz
150ml	¼ pint
175ml	6fl oz
200ml	7fl oz
250ml	8fl oz
275ml	9fl oz
300ml	½ pint
325ml	11fl oz
350ml	12fl oz
375ml	13fl oz
400ml	14fl oz
450ml	¾ pint
475ml	16fl oz
500ml	17fl oz
575ml	18fl oz
600ml	1 pint
750ml	1¼ pints
900ml	1½ pints
1 litre	1¾ pints
1.2 litres	2 pints
1.5 litres	2½ pints
1.8 litres	3 pints
2 litres	3½ pints
2.5 litres	4 pints
2.75 litres	5 pints
3.6 litres	6 pints

TEASPOONS

1 tsp	5g
1 tbsp	15g
1 tsp	5ml
1 tbsp	15ml

OVEN TEMPERATURES

110°C	(225°F)	Gas Mark ¼
120°C	(250°F)	Gas Mark ½
140°C	(275°F)	Gas Mark 1
150°C	(300°F)	Gas Mark 2
160°C	(325°F)	Gas Mark 3
180°C	(350°F)	Gas Mark 4
190°C	(375°F)	Gas Mark 5
200°C	(400°F)	Gas Mark 6
220°C	(425°F)	Gas Mark 7
230°C	(450°F)	Gas Mark 8
240°C	(475°F)	Gas Mark 9